HOW TO LISTEN
SO MEN WILL TALK

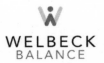

WELBECK
BALANCE

ABOUT THE AUTHOR

Tom Chapman is an award-winning barber, author, public speaker and international educator. He spends his time delivering talks at universities, schools and events, attending industry shows and appearing in the media, trying to reduce the stigma surrounding male mental health problems and suicide – and campaigning for improved mental health facilities and suicide prevention. Tom is a global barber director and has travelled the world cutting hair onstage in front of thousands of people, from LA to Hawaii to Brazil, Australia and beyond.

In September 2015, Tom founded the Lions Barber Collective (LBC), which started as a group of international barbers raising awareness about suicide prevention and mental wellbeing. He believes that the barber's shop is a great, safe place for men to talk.

In 2017, the LBC launched BarberTalk, a training tool for hair professionals across the globe to Recognize, Ask, Listen and Help those in their chairs. From the success of this course, the LBC expanded these programmes, which are now endorsed by Habia (recognized by the UK government as a standard-setting body) and are part of their Continuing Professional Development (CPD) course. Tom has plans to turn the model into a regulated, non-industry-specific qualification that will be recognized globally.

Tom has received a Points of Light award for his outstanding volunteer work from the UK Prime Minister and received a royal endorsement when Prince William requested to meet him in 2019. He is the author of *The Barber Boom* (2018), *BarberTalk* (2019) and a children's book, *The Mighty Lions and the Big Match* (2021). He lives in Torquay, UK with his wife and two boys.

Tom's vision is of a world free from suicide, and to achieve this he is striving to create non-clinical, non-judgemental safe spaces where people feel comfortable to open up and speak about their mental health, and from where they can be signposted to support and information.

Connect with him on Instagram @tomchapman_hair or on Twitter at @HeresTommy.

HOW TO LISTEN
SO MEN WILL TALK

Four Steps to Get Men Talking About Their Mental Health

Tom Chapman

Foreword by
Dr Peter Aitken

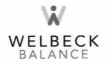

WELBECK
BALANCE

Published in 2022 by Welbeck Balance
An imprint of Welbeck Trigger Ltd
Part of Welbeck Publishing Group
Based in London and Sydney.
www.welbeckpublishing.com

A CIP catalogue record for this book is available from the British Library

ISBN
Paperback – 978-1-78956-292-7

Typeset by Lapiz Digital Services
Printed in Great Britain by CPI Group (UK) Ltd, Croydon CRO 4YY

10 9 8 7 6 5 4 3 2 1

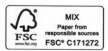

Note/Disclaimer

www.welbeckpublishing.com

To all the grandfathers, fathers, sons, brothers and
those who listen to them

FOREWORD

This excellent little book will give you the tools you need to help someone you know talk to you. It will help you encourage men to work through problems by learning to open up about their mental health – something that, historically, men have struggled to do.

By following the Steps in this book, anyone can learn techniques that will encourage discussion, which is the first step toward healing issues like depression and anxiety.

I am concerned about male suicide. Although still relatively rare, you might be shocked to learn that it's the most common cause of death in men under 49, and is almost twice the rate of women. And I believe we can do so much more to help men who are struggling with their mental health: it begins with a conversation.

Tom and the Lions Barber Collective have paved the way. They show that ordinary people with a little bit of training can do extraordinary things, guiding people through their mental health problems and create open conversations.

Dr Peter Aitken MBChB MRCGP FRCPSYCH DCH DRCOG FHEA
Hon Associate Professor, University of Exeter, College of Medicine and Health
Member, Steering Group, ZeroSuicide Alliance
Former Medical Director & Executive Lead for Suicide Prevention Devon Partnership NHS Trust, UK

CONTENTS

INTRODUCTION

It's likely you've picked up this book because you're worried about someone you know – perhaps a husband, partner, friend, son or colleague. You have noticed that they're down, struggling, anxious – but they also won't (or can't) articulate it. You don't know what to say; how to start the conversation. And you don't want to make things worse, insult or embarrass them.

Men's mental health is a complex – and, at times, intimidating – topic. Alongside a general knowledge about mental health, you're also working against decades of ingrained ideas about what is "acceptable" to talk about and what's not. You're fighting against ideas such as "boys don't cry", "real men don't show emotions" and "it's weak to have a mental illness".

This book won't tell you how to diagnose a mental illness and you will not become a medical practitioner or counsellor after reading it. It is not our place to put a label on someone's behaviour – but the good news is, you don't need to in order to make a difference to someone who is struggling.

What this book aims to do is to enable you to have an impact on the men in your life by giving you the knowledge and tools you need to start and continue conversations in the best, most effective and helpful way. It will help you notice if someone is struggling, suffering or dealing with something, give you the words to ask them how they are, listen effectively and help signpost them to any help they may need.

"You don't need to be a mental health expert to make a difference to someone who is struggling."

Whether it's one particular person that has drawn you to this book or you just want to make an impact and start conversations around how men are feeling, you can be a set of eyes and ears in your community and your social circle. So many problems, if addressed early, can be solved by talking things through and offering support, potentially stopping people from experiencing depression, anxiety or other issues – or even suicide.

You may be feeling completely unprepared for this task, but I am positive that you are actually *already* helping, even if you don't realize it. Just picking up this book is a great first step. Do not underestimate the impact of the small things – a nod of the head, a reassuring look or an encouraging prompt – they often mean the most to the individual. Collectively, those small things will add up to a huge difference.

By sharing the tools to open up conversations, I truly believe that this book could save at least one life. There are some shocking statistics on male suicide, which drove me to start my work in men's mental health – we'll explore this more in Chapter 2. Together, we can help men learn how to talk about their feelings, work toward avoiding mental illness and, ultimately, reduce the high number of male suicides.

Let's make change happen.

"Do not underestimate the impact of the small things – collectively, they will add up to a huge difference."

HOW THIS BOOK CAME ABOUT

This book is based on a Four-Step training programme, originally created by me and inspired by the charity I founded in 2015, the Lions Barber Collective.

I want to start with a bit of history – to put into perspective how and why the charity and training began, and where my desire to further the conversation around men's mental health came from.

My friend Alex took his own life in 2014. When I last saw him, only days before, I was completely unaware that he was struggling so much that he wanted to end his life. For a long while after I heard the news, I was dogged by questions as to why he would do such a thing and what more I could have done. Why hadn't I noticed? Why hadn't I asked him how he was and actually listened to the answer? Would I have known how to react or what to say?

Then I started down the "what if?" spiral. What if I had asked him how he was feeling? What if he had told me he felt suicidal and had a plan? What if something I could have done would have prevented the tragedy?

At Alex's funeral, the crematorium was so jam-packed with all those who had known and loved him that I was among many who had to stand. I was ushered down to the front of the room, to a space next to Alex's coffin, staring back at the room full of sadness. I will never forget that day and the looks on those faces – and that is when I decided I had to do something about it.

I wanted to act, to do something. But I was a barber not a therapist! As a start, I decided to create a hairdressing "look book", and a colleague suggested that all proceeds could go to Papyrus, a suicide-prevention charity. I hadn't even known that there were suicide-prevention charities!

Feeling encouraged by how well the look book was received, I then began looking into what else I could do to help bring an awareness of mental health issues and suicide to my world. I had been a hairdresser for many years and had some great contacts in the industry. So, I founded the Lions Barber Collective with the aim of starting conversations around men's mental health. (The name was inspired by the fact that the look book featured people from England, Ireland, Scotland and Wales, just like the Lions rugby team.) We launched on World Suicide Prevention Day, 10 September 2015, and continued to raise funds for Papyrus. The Lions Barber Collective officially became a registered charity on 19 December 2017, and from there I realized how much more we could do as an industry to promote positive change.

THE "POOR MAN'S THERAPIST"

The more I thought about it, the more I was convinced that hairdressers were ideally placed to do more. The hair industry was in a fantastic position to raise awareness of the issue of mental health and male suicide because it is – literally – hands on with the community. Hairdressers are everywhere, from city centres to tiny hamlets, and are accessible and affordable for everyone. Even if you are bald (which is something I have been asked about on many occasions) you can still come into a barber's shop and treat yourself to a relaxing wet shave. No one is beyond our reach!

A barber's shop is a rather special environment, and that's true around the world – from Devon to New York, from South Africa to Australia. It is a distinctly male preserve and somewhere men feel they can talk about subjects as varied as sport, politics, relationships and religion. That also makes it a place where it is most likely they will sound off about problems they might not otherwise talk about.

Barbers have always been known as the "poor man's therapist". On my first day at Toni & Guy – when I was 18 and new to the hairdressing business – my manager told me to be prepared to be a therapist and be told all sorts of things. How right he was.

"What if we could enable someone to recognize when someone is struggling – and give them the confidence to ask the right questions?"

Hairdressers are often with people through their life journeys, experiencing some of their key moments: first dates, proposals, interviews, birthdays, weddings, anniversaries, birth of children, loss of loved ones, redundancies, miscarriages, addictions, bankruptcies – the list goes on. We are there, we listen and, crucially, we are separate from their social circle. They place their trust in us to make them look fantastic, and often tell us their feelings. This role isn't confined to hairdressers – tattooists, beauty therapists, taxi drivers, doctors' receptionists and many others are in this unique position.

OFFERING A CHANCE TO BE LISTENED TO

After establishing that we were in a unique position, the next step was to make the most of this opportunity. On average, hairdressers listen for 2,000 hours a year, so I realized that if we could train them to actively listen without judgement and with complete empathy, it could make a huge difference.

Then I thought further. What if we could train barbers and hairdressers to be better prepared to *start* these conversations? What if we could enable them to recognize when someone is struggling – through small signs and words – and give them the confidence to ask the right questions? And, finally, what if we could give them the ability and knowledge to signpost those in need of help to the right places?

I knew that giving people the platform to talk and be heard can be life-changing, or even life-saving. I wasn't suggesting turning hairdressers into therapists or psychiatrists, but I saw the potential to bridge the gap between the community they serve and the resources available for those who need them. Out of that idea, I created a bespoke course for the barber–client relationship, with the help and guidance of psychiatrist Dr Peter Aitken: BarberTalk.

FOUR STEPS TO HELPING

The aim of BarberTalk is not to diagnose or give medical advice, but to encourage hair professionals to make the most of the unique opportunity to recognize people who are struggling with their mental health and offer them a lifeline and chance to talk. The course defines Four Steps for barbers to follow to help their clients:

1. **Recognize** that someone is struggling
2. **Ask** the right questions
3. **Listen** without judgement
4. **Help** the individual by directing them to the support
   they need

The courses are bite-sized and delivered in an accessible, not overwhelming, way. It has proved more successful than I could have ever imagined. We have been invited to attend festivals, industry shows and other events, and we've gained a huge social media following.

We have also created a Hair&BeautyTalk version and a non-industry-specific version called HereToTalk. All the training programmes are endorsed by Habia (Hair and Beauty Industry Authority – recognized by the UK government as a standard-setting body for the industry) and recognized on their Continuing Professional Development (CPD) course. I have also begun the journey to turn the model into a regulated qualification that will be recognized globally and one day, I hope, integrated into all hair and beauty qualifications.

And I want to bring the Four-Step process to you. To reach as many people as possible. So, this book uses the tried-and tested structure of BarberTalk alongside the insights I have gained from running this training course. I want to help you take these simple but highly effective principles into your conversations and relationships.

HOW TO USE THIS BOOK

It's really important you work through each Step chronologically. The Steps are designed to take you on a "journey" through your relationship or conversation – from recognizing something might be up, through having the conversation and truly listening to someone, and then getting help.

Do turn to a certain Step if you feel you need to focus on that immediately, for example on getting help, but otherwise please read it from front to back!

I have included activities and chances to reflect along the way (called "Pause for Thought"), to help you put what we're discussing into practice, so it's not just theory.

AUTHOR'S NOTES

I'm very aware that there is a lot of generalization in this book – a lot of "men do this, and women do that". I want to make clear from the outset that I'm aware that the topics of mental health and gender roles are highly nuanced and complex. I do not mean to dumb down this topic, or reduce it to basic stereotypes – however, some general statements about each gender is needed to get the point across. I hope you will forgive any sweeping statements and know that my intention is to impart knowledge and not to further feed the fire of a clear-cut gender divide. Mental illness does not recognise gender, race, religion, borders, age, etc.

Throughout the book I use examples and case studies. These are all based on my experience with real people, although some names have been changed. The advice in this book comes from my extensive lived experience; I am not medically trained. I've tried to keep the guidance as broad as possible to allow the reader to tailor it to the individual in question.

Lastly, before we dive in: a quick thank you from me, for being willing to learn and help further the conversation. It's not easy, it may feel awkward – very awkward at times – but talking really is the best way to bring issues to light!

PLEASE NOTE

If you are concerned about someone you know, and think they may be at immediate risk, please contact your country's emergency services. Details of national helplines and mental health services are also available in Useful Resources at the back of this book.

1

UNDERSTANDING MEN'S MENTAL HEALTH

Before we can begin to meaningfully change *how* we talk to the men in our lives about mental health, we first have to really understand *what* we're talking about.

You may feel that the statement, "Men struggle to discuss mental health more than women" is too sweeping a generalization – but there is evidence to support it. You may be able to think of many of your close male friends or relatives who don't appear to struggle at all. But I'm sure you can also think of many others who would be reluctant to have that conversation and hardly ever show their vulnerable side.

So, before we look at the practical steps you can take to help the men in your life, let's look first at the problem itself.

WHAT IS MENTAL HEALTH?

In order to address something properly, you have to understand it fully. You can't fix a car if you've never looked under the bonnet, and you couldn't write an essay on a book you've never read. So let's first answer a really basic question: what is mental health?

The best way to think about mental health is to think of it exactly how you'd think about physical health. Just as physical health ranges from a slight sniffle or a headache, to more serious problems such as heart attacks, cancer or strokes, our mental health is the same. Sometimes you just feel a little drained, let down or fed up, and that can be minor and temporary. Or you may feel a deeper, longer sense of darkness or despair. Let's face it, the global COVID-19 pandemic that began in 2020 confirmed that we all suffer from mental health issues of one kind or another – whether they are associated with loss, illness, lockdown, home schooling, being furloughed or working on the frontline. Life is hard!

"Our mental health changes from day to day and we all go through peaks and troughs. Life is hard!"

2

Conditions such as anxiety, bipolar disorder, depression, personality disorder and post-traumatic stress disorder are all recognized *medical* conditions. While we cannot (and should not) stray into diagnosis of a person's problem, we do need to be sensitive to the huge array of mental health issues and their ability to affect us all, as well as the myriad solutions available. That should help to dispel the stigma and taboo associated with poor mental health, and to banish thoughtless expressions such as, "That woman is so bipolar!" Or, "That guy is *mental*; he should be locked up!"

Everyone reading this will have been let down, disappointed, not liked themselves momentarily, felt regret, and even felt that they just wanted to escape and hide from it all. This is all completely normal.

We have all had our good and bad days, sometimes with no tangible reason. Just as some days we feel full of energy and other days we can have a headache or a minor injury of some kind, our mental health also changes from day to day. We all go through peaks and troughs.

We will all need help from time to time – and we need to begin applying more sensitivity, and attention, to this topic.

THE DIFFERENCE BETWEEN MEN AND WOMEN

This book is specifically aimed at getting MEN to talk. It acknowledges the (blanket) theory that women are "better at talking about their emotions and mental health than men".

Many opinions on this subject will be shaped by personal experience. For example, you may have noticed a reluctance to talk about mental health from the men in your life – perhaps a dad that never showed emotions, or an uncle that thinks men these days just aren't what they used to be.

To move this point beyond anecdotes – and to show "evidence" of the male struggle with mental health, we will look at some statistics behind this theory. In particular, some shocking statistics regarding male suicide.

Data collected from the offices of national statistics in the UK, Australia and the USA shows the same trend: men are disproportionately more likely than women to take the most extreme reaction to mental health issues – to end their own life.

Breaking it down to look at the number of recorded suicides in 2018, Australia reported deaths of 18.6 males and 5.7 females for every 100,000 people; Scotland and Northern Ireland reported 17.2 males and 5.4 females; England and Wales reported 16.2 males and 5 females; and the USA's results were 22.8 males and 6.2 females per 100,000 people. Significantly more men than women.

Statistics also show that there *appear* to be more women than men suffering from mental health problems: in the UK, it's one in five women compared to one in eight men, and in the USA it's roughly one in four women to one in six men. (But, how would they gather any accurate comparative statistics when so many men tend to suffer silently and alone?) And although more men take their lives than women, women are twice as likely to self-harm. While these statistics are interesting and helpful to know, it's not useful to compare and try to argue that one gender is worse off. Both genders struggle significantly, just in different ways. We need to understand this to best help people.

"Sadly, men are good at hiding their emotions. I believe this needs to change."

I wrote earlier about the flurry of questions that went through my mind after my friend Alex's death in 2014. They can all be distilled down to one word: why? I believe the fundamental answer is rooted in society's idea of what it is to be a man. Men are turning what are perceived as their strengths in on themselves – with fatal results.

Sadly, men are good at hiding their emotions. It is often said by those who are closest to a death by suicide that they didn't realize the person was suffering. This is what I believe needs to change.

Let's look at some of the reasons for that, because if we understand the reasons behind these statistics, we can learn something from them in order to help men cope better.

TRYING TO BE STRONG AND SILENT

Until relatively recently, mental health was not considered something to talk about – for men or women. While anyone would happily admit to a broken leg or a dose of the flu, admitting that you were suffering from depression, anxiety or any other mental health problem was taboo. But as society began discussing mental health more freely, the stigma about men's mental health lingered – far longer than it should have. Men ignored or hid their issues, still fearful of the reproach of their peers or society.

Historically, men are supposed to be strong. They are the hunters, the protectors, dealing with life's dangers without being held back by emotions. When we – both men and women – use words such as "manly", "macho" and "masculine", we are probably not aware of the fact that they carry with them a whole raft of subliminal meanings. Think for a moment about what springs to mind when you read those words. Now think about the *opposite* of those words. What springs to mind then? Weak? Timid? Feminine?

How many boys still grow up hearing "Stop acting like a girl!" or the dreaded "Man up!"? The message behind those phrases is clear: vulnerability and emotional expression is bad, and hiding your feelings and projecting strength is good.

We may not admit to thinking it consciously, but by using that sort of language, even as we hurtle through the 21st century, we are clinging on to definitions laid down when we all lived in caves and hunted with spears, constantly under threat and on the edge of survival.

HOW WE TALK TO OUR CHILDREN

In order to make men feel more comfortable in seeking help, we all need to start well before adulthood. Boys do cry – and why not? – and they should be allowed to feel their emotions. If you're a parent, grandparent, uncle or aunt, or family friend, consider your language around children – show them that emotions are normal and that it's OK to feel bad as well as good.

Our media has always been filled with images of "strong" men – from the stoic heroes of 1940s Hollywood to the muscle-bound superheroes of comic books – and that idea is internalized by boys from a very young age. Strength in men has long been equated with not showing emotion, and that needs to change.

"There is more we can all do to challenge the ingrained social ideas of what's OK to talk about and what's not."

Among this subconscious belief about manhood – and the emotive language surrounding it – is where we may find some answers to our questions.

Thankfully, the conversation around men, masculinity and male mental health *is* now moving forward, slowly. But there is more we can all do to challenge the ingrained social ideas of what's OK to talk about and what's not.

When someone hits a bad patch in their life, whether it's something serious or just those everyday things that can make anyone feel low, what do they do? How do they cope?

First, what do women do? Very generally speaking, they talk about it, they enlist the validation and support of their friends, they share their emotions, they ask for help.

> "You may have heard of men talking about 'admitting' to feelings of depression or other mental health issues, as though it were something to be ashamed of."

What do men do? When men hit a downtime in their lives, they so often add to their own problems by acting in the way they believe men *should* act: strong and silent. There is a stigma around a man admitting to anyone that they are feeling crap and don't know what to do about it, and an almost absolute taboo about asking for help. This can lead some men to reach for drink or drugs as a form of self-medication.

When a man's mental health hits a low point, those social pressures make it a difficult, sometimes impossible, subject to speak about. You may have even heard of men talking about "admitting" to feelings of depression or other mental health issues, as though it were something to be ashamed of.

LETTING SHAME STOP US ASKING FOR HELP

Let's look at an example, and I'll make it *extremely* stereotypical for clarity! Imagine being a tall, muscly, tattooed construction worker who is greeted on site by the usual, "All right, mate?" What would happen if you told your workmates you were feeling vulnerable and depressed? Do you think you'd get the support and response you'd need? It's doubtful.

I used to live with some guys who worked in construction – a world that couldn't be much further from cutting hair! – and saw these "emotional barriers" first-hand. That kind of stigma in a hugely male-dominated environment may have something to do with the construction industry in the UK having the highest rate of suicide, with more than one a day.

Is it this fear of showing weakness among their peers that causes men not to talk about their mental health? It would seem so, but there is more to it than that.

BREAKING DOWN THE FEAR OF NEGATIVE REACTIONS

Dr Brené Brown has conducted extensive research on the topics of shame and vulnerability, which is documented in her fantastic book, *Daring Greatly* (Penguin Books, 2015). She found that not only do men fear opening up to other men about their struggles and emotions, but there is also a huge fear of opening up to the *women* in their lives, too.

Historically, men might have worried about telling the women in their lives about their mental health issues because they believed women genuinely wanted to see them as strong and not weak. I am sure that, with the expectations previously placed upon men, it must have been difficult for those who saw the men in their lives as the "head of the household", the family's "rock" or "strong one", to then have that man break down and tell them they're not coping. It would have been difficult for both parties.

Those same men may have felt they'd be judged for showing any emotion at all. Being laughed at for crying at an emotional film, for example, may have caused someone to close back up, worried that any further display of emotion would be similarly ridiculed.

While some men may still feel like that, and some women still have those expectations of men, that way of thinking is increasingly becoming a thing of that past. Thankfully, men feel more comfortable showing their emotional side – as Brown's research shows.

Over and over in the interviews she conducted for her research, Brown heard men talk about how women were constantly criticizing them about not being open, vulnerable and intimate, and how women were begging to be let in, to have men expose their fears.

> "Your response to vulnerability is so important, as a negative reaction will almost certainly shut a man down."

But when the men responded by admitting to their vulnerability, some of the women's responses to the men in their life were genuinely pretty awful – maybe not intentionally, but they clearly demonstrated that they were not ready to embrace a man's vulnerability, or they were not prepared to respond well. This response is so important, as a negative reaction will almost certainly shut a man down.

"When men got brave enough to [open up], the message they received from the women in their lives was, 'I can't stomach your weakness.' When men dare to be vulnerable, women often recoil with fear, disappointment and disgust, sending men the clear message that they better 'man up'."
Brené Brown, *Daring Greatly*

Both men and women must come to terms with the truth of the situation: men experience emotion as much as women do.

Because of this societal pressure, men have become very good at always pretending to be fine. They can be so good at it, in fact, that if they finally end their own life, even their closest friends and family will be deeply shocked. (This can often be the case for female suicide, too.)

If we're going to start, and continue, these crucial conversations, we must understand where any reluctance to open up comes from, and how we can address that. We'll talk about creating a safe space later in the book.

WHY MEN DON'T SEEK HELP

Many men won't go to their doctor for their physical health, let alone their mental health. They tend to hope an issue will just go away.

When was the last time the man you want to help went to see the doctor? Had they met that doctor before? Compare that with how often they have visited the barber. Do they see the same one each time? I cannot guarantee the answers, and I'm writing from a British point of view, but I bet for most men they've seen the barber more times than the doctor in the last 12 months.

As there is no longer the old-fashioned family doctor, there isn't really much of a relationship between a man and the healthcare system. Could this distant and damaged relationship with healthcare be part of the reason why men don't seek help when they need it?

Only one in eight adults with mental ill health in the UK are currently seeking treatment, and that's mostly in the form of medication. In the US, the figure is slightly better, at a little over one in three.

"We need to begin building bridges between men and the resources available to them."

In the UK, males make up only 36% of referrals to the Improving Access to Psychological Therapies programme. Half of those who die by suicide are not in contact with any mental health services and are, therefore, completely unknown to the system. The official figures from the National Confidential Inquiry into

Suicide and Safety in Mental Health (NCISH) state that 72% of all people who take their life have no contact with mental health services in the 12 months beforehand.

Men need to take more responsibility in seeking help when they need it, and that's built on confidence. What *we* can do is start conversations and begin building bridges between men and the resources available, giving them the confidence to reach out and reducing the stigma for those accessing them.

These avoidant behaviours are imprinted into the male psyche and are really hard to change. I spend my life working in mental health and even I'm guilty of avoiding the doctor!

COMMUNICATION AND LONELINESS

An important contributor to the prevalence of mental health issues is the break-up of the social fabric that has occurred in the last several decades. Even though we may live in close proximity with others, they often remain strangers, and there are many people suffering alone who have no one to turn to.

In 2018, a Minister of Loneliness was appointed in the UK – that's a dreadful admission of our failure to communicate!

We thrive on human connection, and anything we can do to make connections with other people will benefit all of us.

We all need to love and be loved, as well as to belong – these are basic needs of the human condition.

You've already made a big step toward addressing the problem by picking up this book. You're making sure you're there for someone when they need you, and that cannot be undervalued.

WHAT CAN HAPPEN WITHOUT HELP

Men tend to keep everything bottled up inside and do nothing. But doing nothing is not a viable option, because while our moods go up and down, mental health issues do not necessarily go away by themselves, and the more serious they are, the less likely it is that they will go way of their own accord.

By not being treated for their mental health, or not even recognizing it as a problem, men struggle alone and can end up in seriously low states of wellbeing (and mental illness) before they are even aware of it. Once in that space, it's hard to get out alone.

Often men will resort to self-medication or escapism in food, drugs or alcohol to try to cope with these issues. Take a look at some startling British statistics from the Mental Health Foundation:

- *Men are more likely than women to have an alcohol or drug problem. 67% of British people who consume alcohol at 'hazardous' levels, and 80% of those dependent on alcohol, are male.*
- *Almost three-quarters of people dependent on cannabis and 69% of those dependent on other illegal drugs are male.*

And, as we touched upon when looking at evidence for this problem, male suicide rates show what can happen if mental illness is left untreated. You may have heard the statistic from the UK that if you are male and under 45, you are more likely to die of suicide than anything else. That's a sobering thought. And globally, 75% of suicides in the UK and Australia and 79% of suicides in the USA are men. I believe we can change these statistics.

My hope is that the tools in this book will enable you to help someone you know, and make that difference.

TALK ABOUT YOUR OWN MENTAL HEALTH

I do believe the stigma attached to problems such as depression is being worn down, especially when people talk about their *own* problems.

There are huge numbers of men (and women too) with a high media profile who have been open about their problems with depression: Brad Pitt, Hugh Lawrie, Dwayne Johnson, Stormzy, Bruce Springsteen, Kid Cudi and Donald Glover – to name a few. Their bravery goes a long way to break down stigma.

The more people – especially men – share their stories, the more it should encourage men to open up and acknowledge their issues.

So, please do start sharing how YOU are feeling – especially if you're a guy!

WHAT CAN WE DO TO SUPPORT MEN'S MENTAL HEALTH?

The good news is that things are changing in the conversation around mental health. Men are increasingly being encouraged to throw out the outdated macho stereotypes and talk about how they are feeling. Counselling services are becoming more available and their use normalized.

There is still a long way to go, but I have seen for myself that changes are happening in the younger generations. When I held a pop-up barber's shop with the Lions Barber Collective at some British universities, the students were very keen to open up and talk about their mental health – some before we even talked hair!

PREVENTION IS BETTER THAN CURE

The old saying that prevention is better than cure springs to mind time and again when talking about mental health, and surely prevention is the most preferable option.

I was once told by a therapist that the premise of BarberTalk is so effective because we are dealing with issues before they become serious. We are there, asking good questions and actively listening to those in our barbers' chairs, and as a result people feel sufficiently comfortable to offload their worries and concerns and just let off steam.

She went on to explain that by the time people get access to her, their issues may have worsened – and in the worst cases they may already have lost their job, their family, their home and could even be struggling with addictions. Once they have reached that point, they have a mountain to climb to get themselves out of the situation they are in.

"Starting a conversation may take some courage on your part, but it will be worth it. After all, what's the worst that can happen?"

LEARN TO LISTEN

This is where this book comes in. Learning to listen to men and encouraging them to talk about their feelings is something we can all do. BarberTalk started in barbers' shops because I happen to be a barber and was ideally placed to offer a listening ear to our clients. But it doesn't matter who we are or what our relationship is with the person in trouble – the idea of this book is that it extends beyond the salon and into society in general. The skills outlined in this book are for everyone to help anyone – partner, husband, father, son, friend, colleague or even a stranger – and the more people who learn to use these skills, the more men we can help.

You will have many opportunities every day to establish communication with men in whom you recognize a potential problem. It may take some courage on your part, but it will be worth it. After all, what's the worst that can happen?

When we stand a chance of recognizing the signs that someone may be struggling, it should give us the confidence to ask the right questions and combine that with the ability to listen well, actively, without judgement and with plenty of empathy.

By intervening at the earliest possible moment, we can make a huge difference.

Yes, we can hopefully reduce those shocking statistics, but we can also just start some helpful conversations and make someone's day better – it doesn't have to be any bigger than that.

Let's look at the Four Steps and how to have those conversations.

2

GETTING STARTED WITH THE FOUR STEPS

Using the training framework that became BarberTalk, I've distilled the process of having a conversation about mental health into four parts. We are going to explore four different areas of communication, which take you through the process of getting a man to open up about mental health issues and guiding him toward the help he needs. By progressing through each Step, you will gradually develop your communication skills.

The Four Steps are to:

1. **Recognize:** By observing changes in behaviour – including realizing what *isn't* being said – you can learn to identify a potential problem (more on this later).
2. **Ask:** Begin to ask open-ended, unthreatening questions that may draw out any repressed feelings and create space for reflection.

3. **Listen:** Really listen to every word, and make no judgements.
4. **Help:** Don't offer your own solutions; guide them toward finding their own solutions or signpost them to where they can get appropriate help.

The Four-Step process will allow you to offer help to a man you know; the system is flexible enough to allow you to adapt it appropriately to the relationship and the circumstances. In fact, you'll probably find that it generally improves your conversations – after all, who doesn't love that friend who knows just when to let the silence settle and when to jump in with a question?

> "You are not here to 'fix' anyone – your role is just to recognize, value and listen, then let that person know what help is available if they need it."

FEEL THE FEAR AND DO IT ANYWAY

The first thing I am going to ask you to do is to do away with any feelings that you are underqualified for this work (even though I felt exactly that), so it is important to establish exactly what we are trying to achieve here.

After reading this book, there is no suggestion that you are going to be an expert on mental health of any kind – so don't expect your PhD through the post any time soon! The idea behind this method is, in fact, the complete opposite. I don't want people to try to be therapists, psychiatrists, doctors or counsellors. This isn't about diagnosing or prescribing, and that is the beauty and part of the success of the whole thing.

I have spoken to people who have said, "It's not my role to look out for everyone's mental health and solve their problems." I couldn't agree more. That is not what I ask of anyone. You are not here to "fix" anyone – even in the unlikely event that they wanted it. Your role is just to recognize, value and listen, then let that person know what help is available if they need it. It can also be hard to let go of what you've heard or learnt from someone in pain, so we'll look at some coping strategies later in the book.

This non-clinical approach focuses on the human condition, rather than on specific mental health conditions. I am not here to give you a scientific list of what anxiety looks like, or the signs of bipolar disorder or how to diagnose imposter syndrome. That is a job for the professionals, plus this book would weigh about 20kg and I would have epically failed at creating a handbook that can be used by anyone. We don't need to know all that. It's enough for you just to recognize when someone isn't their normal self or seems to be struggling – nothing more than that.

Another common fear you might have is that you might get it wrong and the person will be offended; or that you won't know what to do or say; or that it will be awkward or the person will get upset. Forget all that. Worst-case scenario: you get it wrong and your initial question is rebuffed. So what? Even if you get it wrong now and then, you have acted sincerely in reaching out to someone and showing them that you care. No one will be offended that you care about them.

PUTTING THEORY INTO PRACTICE

Within each Step chapter, I've included "Pause for Thought" reflection boxes to help you consider how the theory may play out in real life. By the time you reach the end of the book, you should feel confident that you understand what you can do to make a difference.

For those reflection activities that require you to write something down, think carefully about where you do this. While I'm not trying to encourage secrecy between you and the men in your life, if someone found your notes out of context it could potentially be distressing.

PAUSE FOR THOUGHT

How Confident Are You?

Answer the below questions on a scale of 1 to 10, where 1 is "Not at all" and 10 is "Very confident". We'll repeat the questions at the end of Chapters 4 and 6 and on page 165 to check how you have progressed.

- How confident do you feel about identifying someone who may be struggling with their mental health?
- How confident are you about asking questions that will allow someone to feel safe confiding in you?
- How comfortable do you feel talking about mental health struggles?
- How comfortable do you feel talking about suicidal thoughts?
- How good a listener would you consider yourself to be?
- How good is your knowledge of what resources are available to help those struggling with their mental health?
- Do you feel confident that you could make a positive impact on somieone in need?

HOW THE STEPS RELATE

As you progress through the Steps, you will notice that the Four Steps are interdependent, and that at any point during a conversation you'll likely be using more than one. That's why I'll keep circling back and repeating certain parts as we go through the Steps; they are repeated because they have equal importance and relevance at each moment.

Let's look at how the Steps relate to each other, and how the Steps might work in the real world.

- Be observant of those around you.
- Acknowledge that you are a friend not a counselor.
- **RECOGNIZE** when someone has a problem.
- Find a safe place where you feel you can open a dialogue.
- **ASK** open questions to get a conversation going.
- Let them know that you represent a safe space.
- Show interest (**LISTEN**) and ask questions to keep them talking.
- Watch to see if they begin to relax (**RECOGNIZE**).
- Give them space to talk freely, leaving silences.
- **LISTEN** with your full attention and without judgement.
- Continue to **ASK** open-ended questions.

- Don't stop observing their mannerisms and behaviour (**RECOGNIZE**).
- **HELP** them to find the answers they need or direct them to sources of support.
- Maintain contact and keep going through the process.

It really can be that simple.

3

STEP ONE: RECOGNIZE

Step One is to RECOGNIZE that a man you know may have a problem with their mental health.

This is crucial, because if we cannot see that there is a problem or that a man is struggling with some aspect of his life, then the journey never begins. We cannot ask questions, give someone the opportunity to be heard and a space to be listened to, if we haven't even identified that need in the first place.

By establishing this first step, that then allows us to start using the skills of observation and empathy.

In this chapter we will look at ways of identifying when something is wrong. What are the signs to look for? What methods do people use to hide their problems?

It is often said that a certain person was the "life and soul of the party", and that no one realized they were going through a tough time until it was too late. Does that mean we were too close to them to recognize the markers, or that we were not looking? It could be both – and men can be *really* good at masking their feelings.

There is also the fear of not knowing what to do if we were to identify a problem, and that can make us close our minds to recognition in the first place. Although you've already begun to tackle that fear by reading this book. It's worth keeping in mind that the problem you *think* someone is having might be different or worse than you expect, so try not to assume anything at all at this stage.

"I want to dispel the idea that it is difficult to recognize someone's struggle, when it really can be very simple."

OBSERVATION

A key part of the first step is to be observant. Try not to focus on yourself, but rather watch and listen to those you want to help, and to the men around you.

This has the added bonus of giving you more insight into other people – and imagine how great the positive impact would be if we were all looking out for each other!

SIGNS OF A POSSIBLE PROBLEM

Recognizing when someone has something playing on their mind or is struggling with difficult emotions is a skill that can be acquired with practice. Part of this will come from understanding that mental health issues aren't the cliché they're often portrayed as.

Some of the signs we will look at below may seem obvious, others are more subtle. Most of all, they may be hidden in plain sight, disguised by behaviour we don't associate with depression or anxiety.

What signs are we looking out for? Here are a few examples.

SELF-CARE

- Yawning or looking tired, as if they are sleeping too much or not enough
- Gaining or losing a lot of weight over a short period of time
- Looking unkempt and not bathing or observing personal hygiene
- Obsessing over how they look

BEHAVIOUR

- Being over-animated and speaking loudly and frantically
- Biting their nails or fiddling with their clothes
- Being quieter and more refrained than usual
- Being uncharacteristically late for meetings, events or gatherings
- Being unreliable, or even not showing up any more
- Drinking too much
- Taking drugs or "partying" more than usual
- Stopping gym visits and getting out of shape
- Fidgeting or not making eye contact
- Spending copious amounts of time at the gym to the point of being obsessive
- Isolating themselves
- Stopping engaging with hobbies

I know what you're thinking: "*He's literally listing everything that anyone could ever do, and then also describing the complete opposite! How the hell is that making it easier to recognize that someone may have a problem?*"

And actually, that's really the point, because I want to dispel the idea that it is difficult to recognize someone's struggle, when it really can be very simple. Let me explain.

LOOKING FOR UNUSUAL CHANGE

Essentially what we need to look out for is a *change in behaviour*. That's it! That skill alone will help you protect those in your life, the ones you love and the ones you meet.

It is often easier to spot changes in those we see less often, because changes can appear so gradually that we don't notice them in those we see regularly.

For those we see less often, any change will be more noticeable, as the person's behaviour will contrast to the previous time we saw them. It's just the same as your auntie exclaiming, "Haven't you grown!" when she came to visit when you were a kid.

I see my hairdressing clients every four to six weeks, and many of them have been coming to me for years. If someone living with you gained or lost a few pounds a week, you may not even notice. If my client comes to me having lost a significant amount of weight since I last saw them, I am going to notice that for sure. This can be the same for any other kind of change. And that's why honing your observation skills is so crucial.

PAUSE FOR THOUGHT

Initial Concerns

- Think about someone who you feel might need help.
- What has caused you to have an initial concern?
- Think about any behavioural changes you have noticed.
- Write down in a notebook the main things you have noticed and why you think they are important.

If you're thinking that sometimes people *do* change without any deeper issues, you'd be right. But if you do recognize a change, this is your opportunity to move on to the next Step and ASK that person a friendly question – who knows, it may turn out to be a life-saving question.

There may be a simple reason for the change: New Year resolutions, someone winning the lottery, welcoming a new grandchild or landing a dream job would all be good reasons to act out of character! But if they brush it off, ignore it or try to justify or explain away their behaviour without a convincing reason, then you may have spotted a marker that is worth pursuing.

Let's look in more detail at the all-important areas where you can recognize problem signs.

BODY LANGUAGE

When we communicate, just 7% of the thoughts and feeling we express are through words. Of the rest, 38% is through tone and 55% is through body language, so we need to pay attention to these non-verbal signals that suggest a guy might be going through a hard time.

Let's think about the obvious things to look for that you might associate with someone who is feeling down: slouched, quiet, no eye contact, insular, head down. This is the ultimate expression of someone down on their luck and potentially mentally unwell.

Then there's also those who are frantic, alert, fidgeting and loud.

"Those are the complete opposite of one another!" I hear you say, and you're right, but both are signs that someone may have experienced something to knock them off kilter. Someone may be so terrified of their issues being detected that they overcompensate when trying to hide it.

The key to this, again, is the *change* in that person's behaviour. If the person you know is always a little slow to speak, softly spoken, slouchy and generally pretty reserved, and then all of a sudden they're quite frantic, outspoken, loud and running around the office chatting to everyone, that is a sign something has happened. And vice versa.

It is the all-important change in behaviour. Even if the behaviour they are now showing may be considered as a positive trait in your society, community or workplace, it could be a negative sign toward the state of *their* wellbeing.

Also, be aware of things like new ticks or unusual habits that those around you have just picked up or started doing out of the blue.

FLUCTUATIONS IN WEIGHT

This is something that may be harder to talk about, although it is not impossible. I know that I'm one of those men who goes to food when I'm feeling down: food is my comforter and therefore damages my wellbeing even further!

Keep an eye out for a change in eating habits – either eating more or less. Look out for changes in clothing or *no change* in clothing (they may be staying in certain clothes all the time because they are the only ones that fit or are comfortable).

In a society that associates being happy with being skinny, losing weight quickly may seem like a positive to some, but it can be a sign of desperation or being truly miserable or stressed.

A gradual weight gain or loss could perhaps be explained by lifestyle changes, but an extremely quick gain or loss can be quite serious, both mentally and physically.

The person might joke about their weight and this may come across that they are comfortable with the situation, but it could also be a cry for help. (Keep in mind that a sudden, unexplained weight loss can be a symptom of a physical problem too, such as type 2 diabetes.)

You obviously don't have to mention someone's weight to them when reaching out, but it can be telltale sign that it is time to ask a question about their wellbeing.

CHANGES IN MOOD

I bet you can guess by now what I am going to say. You got it! They could be over-happy or incredibly sad, or anything in between.

Again, if it is a change from their normal behaviour, something may have happened. If it is a serious change in their behaviour and mood – a very deep depression – then we must act on it quickly, and seek help.

Some people are just generally more positive than others; and some people like a good moan. And that's all fine. It's a *change* in someone's personality or general mood that you are looking out for.

Remember: we may associate happy people as safe and in a good place, but those who are struggling are often very good at putting on a brave face so that no one suspects their problem.

WHAT THEY SAY

While you are observing someone and *how* they're acting, you will also need to be attentive to *what* is said. We'll talk later about how exactly to have a difficult conversation, but while we're discussing signs someone may need help, here are a few phrases that may flag an issue.

- *"I've had enough of this."*
- *"I can't go on any more."*
- *"There's nothing to look forward to."*
- *"They're better off without me."*

- *"There's no hope."*
- *"What's the point?"*
- *"I always do everything wrong."*

These are pretty serious statements when you think about it, and most are pretty final. Something like, "There's nothing to look forward to" shows real desperation, because most of us do have *something* to look forward to, even if it's just your date night, a takeaway at the weekend, a glass of wine when the kids are in bed, your favourite TV show, the gym, a meeting with friends or a day off. Generally, there is always something to look forward to.

It's probably unlikely that someone will say these things to you with no context – these phrases will probably pop up after you have observed, recognized and started a conversation.

Remember that these phrases could be thrown out there in mid-conversation, possibly out of desperation. In this case they should most definitely be picked up, as they indicate that the person is feeling strong enough or comfortable enough to reveal their true feelings in that moment. Most of us have probably heard someone say these things in the past but maybe didn't see them as a cry for help or a cause for concern – this is not meant to worry or concern you, but only to ensure we are aware of them in future conversations.

These phrases may take you by surprise, and that can be an incredibly difficult thing to deal with. Thank them for being honest and to ask them why they are feeling that way – there's more on this in Chapter 5, Step Three: LISTEN.

The person may also say what appear to be positive things, such as:

- *"I finally know what to do."*
- *"Things make sense now."*
- *"I have some clarity."*
- *"It'll all be fine soon."*
- *"I have a plan to end the problem."*

Although these seem to be positive at face value – and more often than not, they may well be – they can also be the words of someone who has decided that ending their life (perhaps even ending their life) is the answer to their problems.

Be sure to ask them about the decision they have come to while inviting them to expand and tell you more.

OBSESSIONS

We all know someone who we would describe as "obsessed" with something, and that is normal for them. They love it, live for it and thoroughly enjoy it, and that's fine.

However, if there is a sudden new obsession in a person's life, it may signify a difficult event or some other trouble.

You might know someone who's gone from checking football scores only occasionally to checking them compulsively. Maybe, at the same time, their spending habits have changed or they've become more secretive. This behaviour may lead to – or be caused by – something more serious, and may be an opportunity for you to ask a question to see what has bought this on.

Obsessions can be about many things – from the more obvious ones such as exercise, food and cleaning, to things that you might not think relevant – binging on reality TV, constantly checking football scores or Googling the weather. You are looking for new interests that seem to consume them.

PAUSE FOR THOUGHT

Obsessions or Fixated Behaviour

- What different kind of obsessions can you think of?
- Have you noticed any new behaviour or strong interests in the man you want to help?
- What could this signify?

MOTIVATION

Again, this can manifest in various ways, but, as always, we are looking for a change in motivation that might be rooted in a negative experience.

If someone who is usually raring to go, hitting targets, getting up early to read or exercise and generally progressing forward suddenly has no motivation then that is a pretty blatant sign that something is not quite right. This may be a sign that your work colleague or employee may be going through a hard time or dealing with something troublesome.

Poor mental health can also show up as a friend having no motivation to meet you for that walk or to go for coffee or other social event, cutting themselves off from their normal social circle. This, in turn, can lead to isolation and loneliness, which is particularly dangerous for anyone's wellbeing, particularly for someone who is already feeling low.

On the flip side of this, if someone who generally lacks motivation has started listening to motivational coaches every day and quoting pop psychology at everyone frantically, this too may be a sign that a question may need to be asked (with a kind ear to follow).

SLEEP

Sleep is a funny one. I have two boys of five and three, and they will never admit to being tired, ever! Even when they are lying in bed, fighting sleep with all their might, they will try to come up with reasons to stay up for just another couple of minutes. On the other hand, adults will often compete with each other over who is the most tired!

Adults generally recognize the importance of sleep and it can be a crucial factor in reflecting someone's health. Of course, there are occasionally obvious reasons for staying awake all night: we all know the feeling of lying in bed worrying about something we have to do the next day, or not being able to sleep because we are *so* excited at the thought of picking up a new car or meeting an old friend. (It's amazing how close anxiety and excitement are to one another, isn't it?)

But a constant lack of sleep is a hindrance to our wellbeing, both physically and mentally, and insomnia can create a vicious cycle that can take its toll. A lack of sleep manifests itself physically and it's very easy to spot (you know when someone looks tired!), so this is a good one to watch out for.

At the other end of the sleep spectrum, if someone is struggling to get out of bed, sleeping during the day and is still always exhausted, then there may be something serious going on. They may start to miss events, both work and social, or avoid doing anything active, and just want to sleep all the time. This is just as worthy of attention as someone who isn't sleeping.

LIFE CIRCUMSTANCES

It's always worth remembering that situations that some people may handle with ease may be devastating to others. These difficult life events might show as physically visible signs, as the worry may result in lack of sleep, over- or undereating, a change in body language or an obsession.

Debt, for example, could play a massive role in in damaging someone's mental wellbeing and is something that can easily spiral out of control. You may be able to recognize debt problems if someone has recently purchased a lot and then suddenly stops doing anything that involves money. Perhaps they may avoid the conversation or get edgy when money is brought up.

Other circumstances could be big life events like birth, death, marriage and divorce; worries about children; or an addiction such as drink, drugs or gambling. Sometimes people will bring these issues up in conversation, maybe to test the water. If they do, recognize this as a sign that they would like to offload, and try to give them that platform.

Life circumstances can also be hidden really well, so they may be harder to notice. Maybe they become secretive about where they have been or where they are going. Many people will feel that their private lives are nobody else's business, and will believe they need to fix it themselves. If you know the person reasonably well, then you will have a better chance at noticing if someone is trying to cover something up, but keep in mind secrecy is possible to achieve by anyone.

TOO BUSY TO NOTICE

Recognizing change is really important and it's the initial Step in helping someone in need, so why is this alertness not just "normal" behaviour for us?

We may not recognize some of these signs because we are just too busy, distracted by all the things we try to pack into our lives.

> "We must be curious, and not brush off a change in behaviour as nothing."

Take notice if your son starts spending all their time in their room or alone; or if your housemate's behaviour has changed in some way and they are avoiding company.

Has a friend found excuses not to meet up for a beer? Is your partner more tired and less energetic than usual? We must be curious, and not brush it off as nothing.

However, we may choose to remain unaware because we don't know what to do when we *do* notice someone's change in behaviour. We've never been taught how to talk to someone, and we can be scared: scared we will say the wrong thing; scared that we may make things worse; scared that we cannot solve the problem or fix what is broken; scared we may be the problem; scared that they may be in a bad place or even suicidal.

It's a cliché, but the phrase "ignorance is bliss" rings true here. In these situations, we may panic and ignore it altogether, hoping it will all go away or that they will "get over it" – time being a good healer and all that. This is a defence mechanism to keep ourselves safe and not get involved in something we cannot handle or would feel out of our depth dealing with. We may make excuses to ourselves or justify that we didn't notice.

I can think of occasions in the past when someone has had the strength to open up to me or throw out a comment to say they were struggling, even if it was just to vent. In those situations, when I was younger and didn't know what I do now, I remember either shrugging it off with an awkward, "You'll be all right, mate", or suggested going out for a drinking session – probably the worst idea, given how drastically alcohol can affect mood and behaviour!

I probably said things that I thought were empathetic but, on reflection, were probably more patronizing. I look back now and wish I could have done better, but we cannot change the past. What we *can* do is understand what we could have done better and use that awareness now.

PAUSE FOR THOUGHT

Making it Personal

- Turn your thoughts to the specific individual you had in mind when you bought this book.
- In a notebook, make a list of the potential indicators that you feel that person has shown. You should be thinking about changes to their behaviour.
- Then, fill in some detail about how the signs are expressed in their case, compared to their normal behaviour. Be careful to keep this list somewhere safe – it could be damaging if the man in question found the list.

PASSING THE BATON

If you feel that someone is struggling and needs to talk, but is unlikely to confide in you – for whatever reason – or you feel you don't have the skills or knowledge to cope with a conversation with this particular person, you may want to consider other options.

Think about the dynamics of your relationship with this person and be honest with yourself. It does not mean you have not succeeded; it just means that you need to look at alternatives. There will be people in your life who you'd feel more comfortable talking to than others – that's just life!

If you find yourself in that situation, what you should not do is assume things will work out in the end and so do nothing. You have accepted a responsibility in recognizing a potential problem, and you can still do something to help.

Ask yourself who this person *would* trust enough to talk with. Do you know of a friend or colleague of this person that you could talk to in confidence? If so, it may be the time to tag that person in – providing they're willing, of course.

Think about how you are going to open the conversation. Where should it take place? Would it be better in person or over the phone? At work or in free time? Be straightforward about what you have noticed and why it has concerned you. Don't elaborate, especially not with conjecture.

For example, you might say, *"I'm not sure whether there is a problem, but they haven't been themselves recently and told me that they are struggling to sleep. I know you're his friend, so I just wanted to let you know."*

Hopefully, that person will take on the task of asking a question and looking for ways to help them find the support they need.

So the person you've asked to help out doesn't feel overwhelmed, you could share with them some of the resources available at the end of this book – or you could even give them a copy!

However, just as we have to be mindful of our own mental health while helping a loved one, we also have to be respectful if someone doesn't want to help; they will have valid reasons for doing so.

CONTINUE TO RECOGNIZE

The one main takeaway from this chapter is to remember that it's a *change* in behaviour that we're looking for.

Now we've recognized that someone might need help, we've reached the scarier part: having the conversation itself. The next two Steps will give you some ideas about how to ask great questions, how to listen and how to continue the conversation.

STEP ONE: RECOGNIZE

Once you move on to the next Steps, you should not stop observing and recognizing signals. As you ask questions and give the person time to speak and listen in return, you must always be taking in their words and mannerisms; the recognizing continues throughout the Four-Step process.

4

STEP TWO: ASK

You are now better equipped to RECOGNIZE the signs that someone may be struggling with something in the moment – or perhaps has more serious mental health issues.

However, there is little point identifying someone who may be in need of help if you do not take the opportunity to actually help them! So now it is time for the next stage: creating an opportunity to help by feeling confident enough to ASK a question.

If we are going to help people, we must recognize that, in general, there is a particular set of requirements most people need in order to begin to talk about how they are feeling.

FEELING SAFE

"Fundamentally, it is about feeling safe,
and if someone does not feel safe, they
will not share their problem."

They may, for example, feel able to open up in a barber's chair more easily than to a close friend or partner. In the same way, a son may not want to speak to his parents, or may prefer one parent to the other. This can be for all sorts of reasons: personality, past relationships, fear of disappointing.

Fundamentally, it is about feeling safe, and if someone does not feel safe, they will not share their problem, even if it is something that has been running through their mind constantly for a long time and is keeping them awake at night.

To feel safe, they need to answer "no" to all these concerns.

- *"Will they judge me?"*
- *"Will they laugh at me?"*
- *"Am I being stupid?"*
- *"Does it matter that it doesn't concern them?"*
- *"Will they think I am a burden?"*

- *"Are they too busy to be worried about me?"*
- *"Will they be angry?"*
- *"Will they ignore it because it's not their problem?"*

It is our job to create a safe space – both physically and metaphorically – so that they can open up to us. It's worth noting here that this is a two-way street – you also need to feel safe enough to have that conversation. If you don't, try suggesting a place or time that you feel would work for you both.

FINDING A SAFE SPACE

When you are observing people and hoping to start a conversation, providing a safe space is incredibly important. In my case, I already have my client seated in my barber's chair, a place that represents trust, intimacy and often a long relationship. Even if I am being paid to hold a razor to a man's throat, they still find it a relaxing and enjoyable experience. That is something quite unique and special!

The qualities you are looking for in your safe space are simple.

- They need to feel comfortable and as physically relaxed as possible.

- You want the man to feel they can talk without broadcasting their problems to the whole room.
- It sometimes helps if you are seated next to each other rather than opposite, so that you don't have to make as much eye contact in the first instance.

You will need to find your own safe spaces at home, at work or out socially, and suit them to the person and to your relationship with them.

IN PERSON OR VIA MESSAGE?

Undoubtedly, the best way of having these conversations is in person. Tone is crucially important, and this is so often lost over email, text or other ways of messaging.

However, if your only opportunity is to converse over email or text, do go for it. Many people feel more comfortable texting rather than speaking on the phone or face to face, anyway. Just be even more careful that nothing is lost or misconstrued. A voice note could be a good option because you can get the tone across, but try to make sure they are alone before you send a voice note that could be heard by others.

If you do text, keep it brief and don't write lengthy messages packed with advice! A good rule of thumb is to always keep your message slightly shorter than the one you have just received, and always end with a leading question. For more, search for #chatsafe. It's aimed at young people, but it's packed with great advice.

If you are talking with your partner, for example, you may be most relaxed at home, or there may be a place that is special to you. For a colleague, there may be a discreet corner of the staff room or a favourite coffee shop. It might be more appropriate to be outside; you could find a quiet bench in the park, or a table outside a café.

SAFE PLACES ON THE MOVE

Men are often better at talking while moving or doing something – getting their hair cut is a prime example. If there is an activity going on, it deflects the focus from both people; there isn't the face-to-face eye contact that can sometimes be uncomfortable or initially be perceived as confrontational – although making swift eye contact later can be a sign that you have established trust.

Another example is sitting in a car. Have you ever had that amazing conversation with a friend while travelling somewhere – when you come up with fantastic ideas, have deep heart-to-hearts or in-depth discussions about all sorts of things, some that matter and plenty that don't? There is something about the activity of travelling side by side, with little eye contact and trust in the driver, that enables us to converse freely with no distractions and the gift of time. This could be an ideal opportunity to start a conversation with a friend or partner.

Have another topic of conversation ready or some music queued up just in case they decide that it's not the right time to talk – as they are unable to simply leave the situation, you want them to feel comfortable no matter what they decide.

There are many other ways in which you can create these safe spaces for such conversations, such as during sport or exercise.

PAUSE FOR THOUGHT

Safe Places or Activities

Can you think of three safe spaces or activities that would be conducive to helping someone open up? If you are thinking of a particular person you want to help, target your answers toward them.

If you find it hard, think first about places or activities that would make YOU feel comfortable to open up or offload, and see if they would be appropriate for the person in question.

What are the important qualities you look for? Are they quiet or noisy? Outside or inside? Warm or cool? Discreet or crowded?

Can you identify some places near you that fit your criteria?

Mechanics, sport and DIY seem pretty clichéd "male" things, but these have been used to great effect in place of traditional support groups to get men together and encourage them to open up to one another without really realizing it! They tend to be far more successful than a traditional set-up where you sit in a circle with all eyes on you, expecting you to open up to a room of strangers.

Of course, we need to remember that we are all individuals, so what works for one doesn't work for another; use your knowledge of the individual to help shape your plan.

DO YOU HAVE TIME?

"Are they too busy to listen to me?" This is a huge barrier to beginning a conversation. Who wants to talk about their emotions to someone who is distracted?

When I recognize something has changed in a client, I have to act quickly, as I only have as long as the haircut takes to strike up a conversation. Thankfully, you'll probably have more time.

It is not generally a good idea to delay things if you have recognized a need to talk, but try to make sure you ask your crucial first question when you know you have time for a proper conversation. It is not ideal if your conversation gets interrupted or cut short just when you have got started.

FEAR OF ASKING THE FIRST QUESTION

You are bound to feel a bit nervous about asking the first question. As we touched on earlier, fear may be holding us back from starting a conversation: fear of offending the other person, fear of saying the wrong thing, fear of looking like an idiot, fear of not being equipped for the answer and not knowing what to do should they confirm that they are indeed struggling and may be at a moment of crisis or desperation.

> "If you find your fear growing, challenge yourself with this question: what's the worst that can happen?"

Remind yourself that the first question will be the most difficult, and you will soon gain confidence. When I started on this journey, I was definitely scared of starting those conversations. However, I now realize that it is an honour and a privilege that people feel comfortable enough to open up to me, even if they don't know me. It is incredibly powerful, and something I'm grateful for.

If everyone had the confidence to be that listener, even to complete strangers, imagine the people we could help and the lives that could be saved by doing something that costs absolutely nothing, and that anyone can do.

If you find these fears growing, challenge yourself with this question: what's the worst that can happen? They may brush you off, change the subject or say everything's fine, even when you can tell it's not. If that happens, you've done all you can – and you've shown that you care. If you think they could be receptive, you could reinforce this by saying something like, "I'm here if you want to talk about anything in the future."

There may be another opportunity when you can try again, or that person may choose to come to you when they're ready, safe in the knowledge that you'll be there for them. You've literally got nothing to lose!

PAUSE FOR THOUGHT

Overcoming Fear

Take a minute and think about the fear of asking someone if they are struggling – the fear of getting it wrong, or the fear that we may not like the answer because our suspicions are RIGHT.

It isn't a nice feeling, being out of our comfort zone. But that moment when you seize the opportunity to ask may be someone's lifeline. It might be the moment you save that person's life.

It is really important to seize that opportunity once you recognize a problem. If in doubt, go back and review the signs of recognition again to give yourself more confidence in these moments.

DEVELOPING A "STOCK" OPENER

So, you have identified that you think someone might be struggling, and you are ready to try to get them to open up.

When we start a conversation, our first question is our opening gambit – it needs to be something that will start a dialogue rather than a deep and meaningful question. Our initial questions are designed to relax the other person and reassure them that they have found both a time and place where they feel safe and a person they feel they can offload to.

It's not a bad idea to have an opening question ready. How many times have you asked or been asked these questions?

- *"How's it going?"*
- *"How are you?"*
- *"How's things?"*
- *"You OK?"*
- *"You alright?"*

These kind of questions require only the most surface-level answer.

How many times have you actually just meant "hello" when you've asked these, and were not actually expecting meaningful answer?

And when you're on the receiving end of those questions, how many times have you thought about how you actually feel before you answer? Did you really mean what you said, or were you giving the stock responses of "Good thanks, you?" or "Not too bad, you?", regardless of the truth of the matter?

That's not your fault or a bad thing; it is something we just do as an extended greeting. It's a habit and it ticks a courtesy box. The problem is that these questions have been asked so many times as we meet people that they have *lost all meaning* and simply get an automatic response.

This back-and-forth can often go on for a minute or so before the real conversation starts, if it ever does!

Let the "niceties" flow, but for our purposes, you will have to follow up on the stock response if the exchange is going to be useful.

It's very unlikely that you would ask a question like, *"How's things?"* and get the reply, *"I'm feeling awful, I just can't go on!"* (Having said that, there are rare occasions when someone is really desperate, and they seize on the smallest opportunity to open up and ask for help. In that case you can move straight into more advanced questions and actions; so it is worth being prepared, even though it is one in a million.)

These greetings are part of our common language, and I'm not suggesting that you drop them. Instead, don't accept their reply at face value, and use them as a launchpad for a better conversation.

PAUSE FOR THOUGHT

When Do You Feel Relaxed Enough to Talk?

Stop and think for a second about the last time someone made you comfortable enough to open up and have a really good, long conversation.

What was the situation and setting?

How did the conversation start and how did it make you feel?

Use your own experiences to give you ideas for questions.

THE POWER OF "SMALL TALK"

While we'll look at how the conversation can progress, it all starts with a great question after a friendly greeting.

Things that we might consider "small talk" – such as asking about family, work and general life – are actually at the heart of our lives and therefore crucial to our mental wellbeing.

If there is something wrong with the family or work, it can have a major impact on us.

Never underestimate small talk and the power it has to uncover someone's mental state, and lead to a worthwhile conversation.

HOW YOU ASK

Of course, what we say is important, but so is how we say it. These opening comments or questions may be things we say all the time, but we need to focus on how we deliver them and the timing.

In the previous chapter, I said that 38% of communication is through tone, which shows how important it is.

We should consider our timing when thinking about our tone of voice. Talking quickly may be interpreted as not having the time for the conversation. So, don't move too quickly with your questions. Allow your companion space to answer, without jumping in with another question if they don't answer immediately.

There are also different implications from the emphasis you put on certain words. Consider the three identical questions below, and the difference the emphasis (in bold) makes to the meaning, and to the expected answer:

- *"**Why** do you think that happened?" (Asking about possible reasons)*
- *"Why do **you** think that happened?" (Asking about their personal feelings toward a situation, not anyone else's)*

- *"Why do you think **that** happened?" (Asking about the situation itself)*

Each emphasis may be right for a certain point in a conversation.

Considering the emphasis you use is another reason not to speak too quickly!

Remember, too, that you should remain non-judgemental, and that judgements are often unwittingly communicated through tone of voice (whether spoken or written). I am sure we have all dashed off a quick email in haste that said, *"Yes, of course I will!"* – meaning *"I'd be delighted to"*, but possibly interpreted as *"Don't hassle me, I'll do it as soon as I can"*.

The right tone can make a massive difference and can let someone know that you are giving them permission to talk.

AN OPENING SEQUENCE

Your role in this conversation will probably comprise you asking a series of questions that put the other person at ease and show them that you are sincerely interested and want to know the answer.

REPEAT AN OPENING QUESTION

"Are you OK?" is a good, simple and straight-to-the-point question, even if it has perhaps been over-used in general conversation. Let's start with that basic question and see how the exchange may go.

"Are you OK?"
"Yeah, you?"
"Yeah, fine, thanks."
Pause

The response is a straightforward one, but if you are observant you may notice that things are actually not OK.

The answer may be mumbled or hurried; the body language may be closed; or there may be no eye contact.

If so, you may want to ask a second time with a different emphasis.

*"**Are** you OK?"*

It may sound ridiculously simple but that may just be enough. All that person may have needed was that small encouragement to offload, confide or say something, conveyed by word, tone and emphasis.

No one ever wants to feel like a burden, and may feel your opening question was out of politeness, rather than a genuine enquiry about your wellbeing. By asking that second time, with more emphasis, you're really showing that you care. Establishing that trust is powerful and shouldn't be underestimated.

CALL THEM BY NAME

Another subtle but significant change to the standard opener is to include the person's name.

Think about when you go to your regular coffee shop, bar or wherever you frequent, and someone uses your name. That feels good, doesn't it? It makes you feel recognized, like you belong, and it grabs your attention.

Think about adding the person's name to that same question. Would that not make you feel that they are really thinking about you and sincerely want to know how you are feeling? Try the sequence again.

*"Are you OK, **Pete**?"*

People often mention that there are others worse off, and this can add guilt to the already negative emotions inside them – using their name makes sure we're focusing on them. There are always people worse off; that's not relevant to how someone is feeling right now.

ADD A WORD OF EMPHASIS

You might even want to add a word of emphasis, such as "really", "actually" or "honestly".

*"Are you **really** OK, Pete?"*

By adding "really", we are showing them that we recognize that they are not themselves and we are, in fact, giving them an opportunity to talk about whatever they may be dealing with, offering them a listening ear and a shoulder to cry on, if need be.

That one word, combined with the use of the individual's name, will make the question significantly more sincere and personal.

BRING IN EMOTIONS

Mentioning emotions means they can't pretend you are asking about whether they're the right temperature or comfortable, or whether you are asking a general question.

It requires that the individual stop and think about the answer, drawing out their emotions and opinions. It also hands them control of where the conversation goes next.

*"Are you really **feeling** OK, Pete?"*

BE TIME-SPECIFIC

This is getting better. Any more improvements we can make? What about narrowing down the time frame?

*"Are you really feeling OK **today**, Pete?"*

*"Have you been feeling OK **recently**, Pete?"*

Focusing the time frame on the present moment or recent past helps the person reflect on their actual mood at the time.

If their mood is fluctuating, they may just brush off the question because they are only feeling down some of the time – they focus in on the OK times and so avoid the question altogether, missing an opportunity.

"OPENING UP" AND DROPPING "OK"

I would add two more improvements to our question:

a) focus on how the person is feeling rather than giving them a yes or no question,
b) try to move away from using the word "OK".

"OK" is just an informal way of saying "satisfactory but not especially good". It already encompasses a general level of dissatisfaction but nothing too bad, which is not necessarily how the person is feeling. It takes it back to being a stock question and answer.

Leaving "OK" out and asking them *how* they are feeling makes sure they give you a personal answer.

Together we have developed this simple opening question, which I believe could be used on a daily basis for the betterment of everyone – so simple but so effective.

"How are you really feeling today, Pete?"

LEADING OR OPEN-ENDED QUESTIONS

After your initial opener, there are plenty of follow-up questions that can help confirm our concerns that this person is not in a good place with regard to their mental health.

However, it is best to keep it simple. What you are looking for is a question that can provide a lead-in to the next question, and the next – sometimes also called open-ended questions.

You may not even have to ask many more questions. Often, giving someone that platform by asking a first great question can be all they need to start talking and offload their problems.

Avoid closed questions, which are those that only require a one-word answer, or offer a choice of answers already supplied. For example, "Are you feeling sad?"

An open-ended question starts with words like **why, how, describe, explain, tell me**. It is a question that draws people out, rather than goes nowhere. You could try:

"Tell me how you are feeling."

"Why did you think that?"

"How did that make you feel?"

"How long has this been going on?"

The questions you ask should convey to the other person that you genuinely care, have time for them and are sincere in wanting to know how they are feeling and what they are going through.

FOR CLOSER RELATIONSHIPS

The opening question we developed on page 74 is suitable for many occasions, but you will also need to create your own additional questions for different circumstances.

If you are trying to begin a conversation with someone very close to you, then this kind of small talk would not fit the bill and you will have to think of a different way to start the conversation. This will vary with each individual, but here are a few principles to guide you.

Your question:

- Should indicate that you want to open a conversation without being too assertive
- Should not be confrontational
- Should be suggestive rather than dogmatic
- Should give the person the feeling that they are in control
- Should reassure them that you are ready to listen and will take what they say seriously.

Some potential broad openers could be: "Would you like to talk about X?", "I've been meaning to ask you about X – how are you feeling?" or "Is this a good time for me to ask you about X?"

START WITH THE REASON

With a close relationship, it may be helpful to begin with the *reason* you are starting the conversation – what it was that you recognized.

Some examples might be:

- *"I've noticed you've been spending a lot of time on your own/you haven't been out with your mates recently. Has anything happened?"*
- *"I'm a bit concerned that you seem to have lost your appetite. Is anything on your mind?"*

- *"I wanted to have a quiet chat with you. Do you have time now?"*
- *"I couldn't help noticing you seemed angry on the phone yesterday."*
- *"You know if anything is bothering you, you can talk to me about it?"*
- *"Is there anything on your mind? You seem a little distracted."*

When asking a question using a reason, be honest about your own concerns but don't try to guilt them into talking.

DON'T JUMP IN WITH BOTH FEET

Remember to start gently to put the person at their ease rather than starting with a heavy question, like the ones below. So please don't ask:

"Are you depressed?"

"Are you feeling suicidal?" (As an initial question, see page 82 for more on asking this question.)

"Do you think you should see a doctor?"

Leave the diagnosis to the experts, and see Chapter 4, Step 4: HELP for how to signpost someone to further help.

CONTINUING THE CONVERSATION

So you've bitten the bullet and asked your first question. Well done!

From there, you need to let the conversation flow, allowing the person to set the direction and prompting with open-ended questions to encourage them to open up. You are handing them the platform to talk while keeping them in a safe space.

Remember to keep your questions open so they are in control of the flow and direction of the conversation; that will make both of you feel comfortable with the exchange. The next questions may include:

- *"Tell me more about ..."*
- *"How did that make you feel?"*
- *"How are you coping with that?"*
- *"What did you do about that?"*
- *"What else do you think you could do to change it?"*

Give them time to think through their answers while feeling safe to do so.

Repeating what they reply calmly is a great way of showing you are listening and that you want to hear more from them. We will talk more about this when we get to Step Three: LISTEN.

PUT A TIMESCALE ON QUESTIONS

Another way of getting to the root of an issue is to put a timescale on the situation. Both of the below questions are useful for gauging where this person is mentally:

- *"What have you been up to since I last saw you?"*
- *"Have you got anything you're looking forward to?"*

The first question will let you know how long this person has been feeling down. Most people instinctively like to share something positive that has happened with them recently and they may even share something they consider negative that has happened since you last met. It could be meeting up with old friends, working too hard, not being well, birthdays or family events. If there has been plenty going on until recently, a lack of socializing may point to the cause of their problem.

The second question – looking forward – will also help to let you know if they are feeling down or really desperate. Again, it may be small things or major events, but we all have something to look forward to, even if it is only a new film you want to see, going to the gym, spending time with your partner, or maybe a family barbecue. It doesn't have to be a holiday, new car, house, marriage, pregnancy or something that life-changing! It can be a small thing in life they enjoy. If they can't think of anything, this may indicate their mood.

PAUSE FOR THOUGHT

Three Questions

Write down three questions that you can carry with you wherever you go, ones that will feel natural for you to use when you recognize an opportunity.

Think about what you have just read and think about how you can add your own personal touch to these open-ended and direct questions to help those around you.

THE LIFE-SAVING QUESTION

Asking someone how they really are may be enough to help your friend or partner – all they needed was permission to have a good rant! The value of that cannot be underestimated.

But there are situations where you may have unearthed something more serious. This is not how most of these conversations will go, but it's always better to be prepared, and I want this book to cover all eventualities.

If someone answers your forward-looking question with, *"Nothing. I have nothing to look forward to"*, then they are clearly not in a good place and their outlook is pretty bleak. No hope can feel like no future.

It may be that, if things are really bad, the conversation reaches questions around suicidal thoughts. It should definitely not be your opening comment or question – however much someone seems to be struggling – but something to have in our back pocket should we recognize the need to use it.

They might use expressions like:

- *"I can't go on."*
- *"What's the point?"*
- *"I've had enough."*
- *"I might as well give up."*

This indicates a serious problem and your response has to be equally serious. Brushing off this kind of statement with the following throwaway statements is not going to help.

- *"`You'll be OK."*
- *"Time's a great healer."*
- *"What you talking about? You have so much going for you!"*

This person has been honest and brave in that moment, and although they may not be thinking about ending their life, they are lacking hope, and without hope they may question their future.

In these situations, we need to step outside our comfort zone. We need to directly ask a life-saving question:

- *"Are you suicidal?"*
- *"Are you thinking of ending your life?"*
- *"Do you have suicidal thoughts?"*
- *"Are you thinking of hurting yourself?"*

DOES TALKING ABOUT SUICIDE MAKE IT MORE LIKELY?

If you ask those questions, does it make someone more likely to try to take their own life? I can tell you categorically that the answer is NO. It is most definitely OK to ask someone if they are suicidal, provided they've given indicators that they might be. It is also OK to talk about suicide, as long as it is in a safe manner. Dr Christabel Owens' research on the subject,

Safe to Talk About Suicide, has proved that it is indeed safe talking about it among family and friends.

Dr Owen's research found that while the media can sensationalize suicide in a way that causes real harm, talking about a loved one who has died by suicide, as long as talked about in a responsible and sensitive way, can have protective factors against further suicide. We know that those bereaved by suicide are at an increased risk in the days, weeks, months and even up to two years after the loss, and open conversation is the best way to remember those no longer with us while supporting those left behind.

She also noted that positive stories of people surviving suicide attempts and subsequently rebuilding their lives can save lives.

ASKING THE HARD QUESTIONS

Clive will always stand out in my memory. In the middle of a busy salon, surrounded by staff and clients, I asked him outright whether he had plans to take his own life. I had known Clive since he was around five or six, which is when he came in for his first haircut, and I had always liked him.

He had suffered bullying and behavioural issues, moved from school to school, and eventually dropped out altogether, although he was never any trouble for me.

I always let him pick the music when he was getting his haircut as he had an exceptionally eclectic taste for such a young lad. We used to speak about all sorts and have a laugh, but he wasn't afraid to say when things were bad either.

One day, when he was about 19, he said in an angry but quiet tone, "I've had enough. Sometimes I just want to kill myself." It took me a moment to absorb what he had just said. With a rush of anxiety and panic for this young man I had watched grow up, I stopped what I was doing.

"Clive, do you really want to kill yourself?" I asked him. Immediately he broke down and cried and told me everything that had brought him to that point.

Having made sure he'd be safe in the immediate future, we met for a walk that weekend and talked for a few hours, at which time he told me he didn't want to die any more. Today, he is alive and doing well – and that is the most powerful thing. All of us have the ability to do this for anyone.

I hope that you never have to ask this question of anyone – especially a loved one or friend – but I also hope that you feel you have the knowledge and strength to ask it if you have to, in the knowledge that it is a perfectly safe question.

Be confident that:

- If that person is not considering suicide, you will not be putting the idea into their head, and

- If that person is considering suicide, then you will have given them the confidence to be able to talk to you about it so you can direct them to get some help. (We'll cover this in more depth later.)

By asking them such a difficult and direct question, you are showing that you care and that you don't want to lose them; and you may well be the first person to even ask them the question.

Many suicide survivors describe that they did not want to die but were looking for a way out of a situation that was intolerable and to which they could not see a solution. It's a way out of their *problems* that they are actually looking for, not a way out of *living altogether*. Remember, 8 out of 10 people who attempt suicide are glad they didn't die.

BE DIRECT

Asking someone if they are suicidal can be posed in many different ways, but it is essential when we are asking this question to be direct.

"Are you thinking of taking your own life?" works, but *"You aren't thinking of doing something stupid, are you?"* definitely doesn't, as it is belittling and too vague. At that moment, they may not consider it to be a stupid choice.

And I would not use, *"You're not thinking of harming yourself, are you?"*, as again this is vague, and these negative questions ("You're not … are you?") might lead the person to give you the answer they think you *want* to hear, rather than the honest answer.

Don't be afraid to be direct.

IF THEY SAY YES

If you ask someone if they are suicidal and they reply with "yes", then you need to know what to do. This spans Steps Two, Three and Four (ASKING, LISTENING and HELPING), but since it follows on from this line of questioning, I have kept this guidance together here.

Firstly, make sure you have understood them correctly. Their response may come in many different ways, and may include:

- *"I finally know what to do."*
- *"I've come to a decision."*
- *"Things make sense now."*
- *"I have some clarity."*
- *"It'll all be fine when it's over."*
- *"I am going to end the struggle/pain/problem."*
- *"I think it's the only option."*

Remember that it is quite common for someone to feel like they cannot go on, want to give up or just hide. This doesn't always mean that they want to take their own life. What they do want is a way out of the situation they are in – and suicide is the ultimate solution.

So treat the situation cautiously. Probe gently before deciding on the right action for the circumstances.

Give them a platform to talk and be heard. This may be the first time they have told anyone just how bad they are feeling. ASKING and LISTENING come before HELPING in the Four Steps. Support can come later; signposting too early can seem dismissive and can potentially shut them down.

Remember to never try to fix or solve their issues by referring to your own experiences or comparing them by using phrases such as:

- *"I know how you feel."*
- *"I understand."*
- *"When I felt like this, I ..."*

This is not useful to the sufferer.

You need to ascertain whether they are actively considering suicide (making plans, with *intent*) or if they are feeling desolate, and hopeless but with no immediate plans (thoughts that do not develop into actions, also known as suicidal *ideation*). As you can imagine, this topic is extremely complex. A simple question to ask would be:

"Have you got any plans to act on these feelings?"

This will help you decide what to do next.

IF YOU BELIEVE THERE IS INTENT

If they are thinking of taking their own life and say they have thought about plans, you may both be feeling that this is a scary time. However, it is important to respond well and try to stay as calm as possible.

It's worth reiterating at this point that you do not have to deal with this yourself. It's a huge responsibility and it can be very emotionally draining. We will cover this in more depth later on, but it's vital that you look after yourself when supporting someone else, and please remember that all the resources listed at the end of the book can and should be used by the supporter too. If you feel you may not be the best person for the task, please read "Passing on the Task" on page 138 for more information.

There are some action points below which will help keep both you and them safe for the immediate future. Your response to someone's disclosure of their feelings and emotions is possibly one of the most impactful things to the future of that individual's recovery – but it's also simple. There are plenty of things we can do to help.

- Thank them for being honest with you and let them know that this environment is safe. Remain calm.
- Never try to "guilt" someone into changing their mind by saying "think of your family or friends". They will have thought of them, but they're desperate. It's also worth keeping in mind that just because friends and family is a reason for you to want to stay alive, it may not be for the sufferer.
- Create a plan with them to keep them safe, instead of telling them what to do. This will be different every time. Ask them if "we" should call a friend, relative or housemate to come and take them home, as you don't want to leave them alone. Seeing if they have a support network is important.
- Ask questions such as:
  o *"What's keeping you safe right now?"*
  o *"What could you do to make yourself feel better about this?"*
- Let them know that you are looking forward to seeing them next time and that you will be there for them.
- Signpost them to more help (Step Four).

It is so important that you include them in the process and help them to help themselves.

However, if you are afraid that they may do something imminently and you have extreme concern, it is absolutely OK to call an ambulance or the police. This is something I have had to do in the past, and I am thankful that I did, as the man is still alive today, and although he wanted to die at that moment, he is thankful he did not.

BEING PREPARED

This has probably been a difficult section to read, and it's horrible to think about having that conversation with anyone in our lives. It's my hope that you'll never have to, but it's far better to be prepared. Remember, talking about this can take a big toll on you, so look after yourself and use your support network/ the resources as and when you need to. For example, the UK charity Samaritans has got excellent resources on its website for a whole range of things, including supporting someone with suicidal thoughts.

If someone discloses that to you that they feel suicidal, and you're there to support them in any way, then nothing that happens from that point on is your fault. I know that's easy to say, and harder to believe. If someone close to you does take their own life, then you must reach out for support. Although we know we can be doing so much more as a society to reduce the number of men who take their own lives, it is important to know that we may not be able to stop every single man from doing so. You will not have failed in any way, and it's crucial to keep that in mind as you reflect on this section.

FROM ASKING TO LISTENING

In this Step, we started out with finding a safe place to begin a conversation, and looked at how to create an impactful initial question. We looked at the kind of open-ended follow-up questions that you could use and the importance of asking after how someone is *feeling*.

We also considered instances where you might need to ask really hard questions regarding suicide, and how to do this.

So, you've overcome your fear and gone for it – asked the question and opened up the conversation. This Step is hard, but perhaps not the hardest. We'll now go on to look at the art of listening. And it really is an art ...

5

STEP THREE: LISTEN

All the Steps are important, but perhaps this one is the most crucial: listening. The reason is that this may be the first – or even the only – chance this person has had to be truly heard.

Listening is a real skill, which we will learn in this chapter. The ability to listen can help us unpack an old saying: "a problem shared is a problem halved". Listening to someone, allowing them to talk, prompting them with pertinent questions, can really help them to come to terms with, or maybe even solve, an issue they have been grappling with, and to find the answers from within themselves.

That's what listening – and, of course, counselling, therapy and psychiatry – is all about.

"Listening allows you to understand how they are feeling, while nudging them with open-ended question will keep them on track and help them to express their emotions."

MOVING THROUGH THE STEPS

Remember that the Four Steps are not separate, but overlap. As you progress from ASKING to LISTENING, you will continue to RECOGNIZE and observe, and you will still ASK the occasional open-ended question to keep them talking and thinking over their issues. As you move into the HELP Step, the recognition, asking and listening are still active; it is an ongoing process.

You are likely to get a different response every time you open up a conversation, so there are no predetermined ways to proceed to this stage.

The important thing is that you allow the man to keep talking. What they say will be determined by just how bad they are feeling.

Listening allows you to understand how they are feeling, while nudging them with open-ended questions keeps them on track and help them to express their emotions.

LET THEM TALK WHILE YOU LISTEN

Conversation is something we all engage in every day – and in many different ways now, thanks to advancing technology. We should never underestimate the power of every conversation to keep us in touch with our family, friends and colleagues.

Generally, in day-to-day interactions, we exchange words back and forth like a ball across a tennis court. We listen until we hear something we can relate to or which we have experienced ourselves, then desperately hold on to our own thought, opinion or story until a pause for breath – even if it is a millisecond – allows us to jump in and explain our version of the story or our opinion.

That's fine for normal conversation, and it is why a good conversation can be so varied and interesting, because you can start talking about work and end up discussing how to pickle onions, or the problem with palm oil, or something you've seen on TV.

For example, imagine you're sitting in my barber's chair, looking sun-kissed and well rested, so I say,

"Wow, you have a great tan! Where did you go?"
"Brazil!" you reply.

Now, from that moment I have pretty much stopped listening because Brazil is one of my favourite places on Earth. I have been there a few times with work, and have some great friends there who have taken me to amazing places, shared fabulous meals with me and created incredible memories. I am now waiting for you to finish talking about your experience – or at least pause long enough that I can jump in and say,

"When I was in Rio, we went to this amazing restaurant on the water that looked out on to the Sugarloaf ..."

And so on, completely cutting off whatever you were saying and making it about *my* trips and experiences. Meanwhile, you are waiting for me to pause so you can jump in and take the conversation in a different direction. It really does have the competitive spirit of a tennis match!

So, what if we change that pattern and try a different style of communication? What if my response was not to talk about my experiences but to listen to yours? I could say:

"Wow! I love Brazil. Tell me what your favourite thing was about your trip."

That takes the conversation in a whole new direction. This is a skill we can apply in everyday life – to everyone's benefit! You simply focus on the other person and ask a question that allows them to tell you what they want to say. See how crucial that could be when someone's opening up about their difficulties?

LEVELS OF LISTENING

There has been much research into the skill of listening and its importance, especially around success in life. From author Dr Stephen Covey (*Seven Habits of Highly Effective People*, Simon & Schuster) to the American motivational speaker Otto Scharmer, many experts have shown how we can break down listening into phases and learn how to use those phases to improve our listening skills on a day-to-day basis, such as in a work or social context.

Some divide listening into four phases or styles, others eight. For our purposes, we will look at the impact of five stages of listening, and discover what we can learn from each. We will consider:

- Level 1: Ignoring
- Level 2: Pretending
- Level 3: Selective (fixer or solver)

- Level 4: Attentive or Active
- Level 5: Empathy

PAUSE FOR THOUGHT

Base Level of Listening

Before we learn a little more about each phase, look at the list above and consider your gut reaction – what kind of listener do you think you are most of the time?
Be instinctive. Be honest!

LEVEL 1: IGNORING

At this basic level, you are not really listening to the person speaking. You're busy thinking about your own stuff, about what to say next, or what you want for dinner, or trying to remember to pick up the dry cleaning.

The person talking can see that you are inattentive at best. You can appear distracted and not present in the conversation. You are likely to be looking elsewhere or paying attention to something or someone else. Your body may be turned away or your arms crossed in a communication barrier.

LEVEL 2: PRETENDING

You are listening to the person speaking but you very quickly make it about yourself when you have the opportunity.

When the person is sharing their experience, you start to refer to your own experience and share things that pop into your mind, triggered by what the other person is saying, taking control of the direction in which the conversation is heading. You are certainly more engaged than at Level 1, but not necessarily with anyone but yourself.

LEVEL 3: SELECTIVE (FIXER OR SOLVER)

You are hearing what the person talking is saying, but you're thinking about ways to *solve* their problem, what they could do to change their situation or how your experience will benefit them. You might start to offer advice or suggest ways in which you think they could fix their issues.

"You are aiming to get the person to explore their own feelings and come to their own conclusions. You cannot impose your solution on them."

This is the level at which most of us function, and it might feel as though it is helpful because you are attentive and trying to be helpful. That might be so if you are talking about decorating the house or finding a dentist – you are supplying information on the topic in question based on your own experience. But if you are talking about emotions, what you are aiming for is to get the person to explore their own feelings and come to their own conclusions. You cannot impose your solution on them; they must find their own solution for themselves.

This level of listening isn't allowing them to open up, and can disempower someone from finding their own answers and from experiencing the benefit of helping and trusting themselves.

LEVEL 4: ATTENTIVE OR ACTIVE

Here, you are actively listening. You are being present with the other person, giving them all your attention, asking questions and enquiring. You might also reflect back to them what you think you heard them say to clarify the information, such as:

"It sounds like you're feeling really under pressure right now."

Reflections such as these will act as gentle nudges to get them to explore their own feelings; they may not have thought about the situation in that way before. It is giving encouragement to explore without providing the direction or the specific map.

In psychology, active listening is used all the time in counselling, training and conflict resolution. The counsellor concentrates fully on what is being said so that they can understand, recall and respond.

SYMPATHY, EMPATHY AND COMPASSION

These three words are often used interchangeably in general discussion, but they actually mean quite different things. It is important to understand how we are using these words in order to reach these higher levels of listening.

In particular, the difference between sympathy and empathy is incredibly important in the listening process. We should always be aiming for empathy if we want to connect with the other person. Here are my (very basic) definitions:

Sympathy means that you feel sorry for the other person's situation or misfortune.

Empathy means trying to emotionally understand what other people feel and trying to see things from their point of view. Essentially, it is putting yourself in someone else's position and trying to feel what they must be feeling.

Compassion combines understanding with a willingness to help.

When I talk about empathy here, it's in the conversational rather than the psychological sense; in psychology, empathy gets even more complicated: "emotional" empathy means you are fully engaged with the other person's emotions –

this is not what we are looking for, because you do not want to be engulfed in such negative emotions.

"Cognitive" empathy, however, is a skill that allows us to perceive and understand how someone else is feeling but to remain outside those feelings, listening quietly and understanding their emotions but staying outside the problem.

LEVEL 5: EMPATHETIC

Empathic listening takes active listening to the next level, as it is a structured listening and questioning technique. As well as actively listening, you are also reflecting upon the other person's feelings and experiences in order to gain an intellectual and emotional understanding of what they are going through. At this level, you are completely attuned to the other person, following their lead in the conversation and making the whole experience about them, not you.

Unlike ordinary empathy, however, while you will understand emotionally how they feel, you will remain outside their distress (see the box above).

When you do have the opportunity to ask further questions, encourage them to speak further about the topic. For example:

- *"How did that make you feel?"*
- *"Please tell me more about ..."*

Remember that listening also involves picking up on the subtleties of tone, emphasis and body language – what is left out as well as what is included. Listen for the pauses and silences between the words and consider the emotions lying underneath.

HIGHER LEVELS OF LISTENING

It can be quite a shock to some when you read about these levels, and if you're disappointed to notice that you tend to listen in a lower category than you'd hoped, you are in good company. But the point of this chapter is not to make you think, *"Oh no, I am awful at listening!"*, but to make you aware of what good listening can look like.

Level 5 is what we aspire to, but even the best listeners can't keep that up all the time – you'd be exhausted and you wouldn't say very much to anyone!

In practice, our listening levels are a moving scale. Sometimes you will be at a level 1 – whether you care to admit it or not – and there's nothing wrong with that; sometimes there is just too much going on in your own life! At other times, you'll switch up and down the scale, such as when you have conversations that bounce back and forth with friends, and those tangents just keep coming until neither of you can remember how you began talking about golden tamarin monkeys.

By being aware of these levels and understanding them, we're allowing ourselves to switch on these listening skills when we need them. We have to recognize that we need to just shut up and listen sometimes – recognize that not everyone needs to know our experience or opinion on what we think is best for them. If we cultivate that awareness, our internal voice will learn to understand when to keep quiet and just listen. The only way to gain this is by practice and experience.

PAUSE FOR THOUGHT

Assessing Your Listening Levels

Consider what level you think you usually listen at (be honest!).

Think of three past conversations that you think you could have used a higher level of listening. Perhaps, on reflection, you realize that you made the conversation about your experience, or gave too much advice.

Now consider three people with whom you'd like to increase your active listening, and aim for a higher level of listening.

Could you apply this today?

HOW TO ACTIVELY LISTEN

Letting people know you are listening is a skill in itself, and all these things combined are key to becoming a pretty good active listener.

- **Pay attention:** This seems like stating the incredibly obvious, but that's what makes it important. We expect someone to pay attention to us when we are talking, even if it is about what you had for dinner or your opinion on the music the cool kids are listening to these days. Think about ways in which you can let people know you are listening. Body language is an excellent way to send signals that you are listening, and even how interested you are in what the other person is saying. Make brief but regular eye contact, nod in recognition of what they are saying, turn toward them and keep your body language open.

"When you hear something you can relate to, it may be difficult to bite your tongue, but keep that for another conversation. Don't interrupt!"

- **Let them talk:** We're trying to construct a great conversation around mental health, and that's all about allowing the other person to talk. When you hear something you can relate to, it may be difficult to bite your tongue, but keep that for another conversation. Don't interrupt! You need to keep those lips sealed, even if you think you have solved their problem, or think you know how they are feeling – most likely you haven't or don't.
- **Don't fill the silence:** Silences can feel uncomfortable, and you may want to rush in to fill them. There will be pauses in the conversation, silences while they explore what they want to say next. Resist the temptation to fill them. Be patient – keeping silent will give the other person the space and ability to go further into the topic and their thoughts on it. Let the silences go on for longer than you would in a normal conversation until they begin to feel quite uncomfortable, then you may need to give a gentle prompt to get things back on track:

- o "You said you found it difficult to talk to your boss. How did that make you feel?"
- o "Can you tell me a bit more about what happened?"
- o "Why do you think that made you feel so bad?"

> "Be patient – keeping silent will give the other person the space and ability to go further into the topic and their thoughts on it."

- **Don't complete their sentences:** It's very tempting, but it's not helpful.
- **Do not judge:** Not passing judgements related to your own morals or beliefs can be extremely difficult, but it is an essential skill if someone is going to open up to you. Your lives don't have to align perfectly for you to understand their troubles and potentially help them.
- **Give gentle nudges:** Ask open questions that encourage the speaker to examine their own feelings.
- **Don't give advice:** This is not the time.
- **Repeat it back:** Clarifying the information that they have disclosed to you is a must in active listening. This will reassure the speaker that you are invested in what

they have to say and are taking it on board. Repeating back what they have just said to you and getting them to confirm it has benefits for you both. Not only do you let them know you care, you are also clarifying back to yourself that you heard them correctly. This gives them the chance to agree with you or maybe go into further detail about how they are feeling. Something like, *"So you're struggling to cope with all these new responsibilities at work, is that right?"* will go a long way to reassure that person you are listening.

- **Don't tell them you know how they feel:** However hard you try, you don't know exactly what they are going through and your attempts to relate may sound insincere, even if they are not. Have you ever been pouring your heart out to someone about anything – a break-up, a tough time at work or the loss of a pet – and that person has responded with, *"I know how you feel!"*. How did that make you feel in that moment? I am guessing something like, *"You have no idea how I feel! How could you understand? My relationship was completely different from yours!"*

That is because we will never know how anyone else feels about anything – never! Even if we try our hardest to empathize, and no matter how similar their experience, that person's experience of the same event will always differ. They have a different view on life because of their journey through life, their upbringing, social circle, job, age, relationships, education, interests, motivations and so on. Instead, say something more like:

- *"I realize I don't know exactly how you feel, but I am here to listen, and I will try to understand what you must be going through."*

LISTENING IN ACTION

I asked a friend to meet me for a coffee after I saw a pretty negative social media post about them. After the usual greetings, I very quickly got to the point and asked, "How are you really feeling today, Steve?" It helped that he already knew I was a safe space and completely non-judgemental, but he went on to tell me everything about a mental health diagnosis he had been given and the fact that he had been waiting 18 months for the treatment/therapy he needed with no signs of receiving it soon.

Steve's way of handling a tough moment was to get out of his house and away from his family to cool off and regain clarity. This came with push-back from Steve's partner, who didn't let him leave as they were concerned for his safety and not knowing where he would be, which only upset

Steve further and made him feel "like a caged lion". He also told me that he loved to draw, which would be the perfect way to help him heal in that moment, but since "everyone else's crap" was in the space where he used to draw, he couldn't do that either.

I just continued to listen, allowing Steve to have silences to reflect and search for what he wanted to say next. If he came to a pause and looked like he was worried he had lost me, I'd encourage him with a comment like, *"Tell me more about why drawing helps."*

Steve went on to tell me about how he owned a small flat with a nice view, but it was a bit of a mess and no one really used it, although him and his partner had talked about cleaning it up and making it a safe bolthole to retreat to. After a good couple of hours of chatting, there was a long pause. Eventually I said, *"When are you going to go and sort out the flat and turn it in to your little studio?"*

By simply listening to him and not rushing the process or looking for ways to fix or solve his problem, I was able to give him the time and platform to get his thoughts out of his head and into his mouth. Just by sounding off to someone who paid attention, cared and gave him encouragement, he was able to solve his own problem.

HOW TO LISTEN EMPATHETICALLY

All the points under active listening apply to empathetic listening, but there is an additional layer to empathetic listening.

- **Be fully present:** You need to be 100% there for the speaker in that moment, forgetting everything else going on in your life or around you to focus completely on the needs of the individual.
- **Empathize with their emotions:** Try to fully understand the emotions they are experiencing.
- **Maintain a degree of detachment:** You must remain outside of their problem.
- **Listen to what they aren't saying**: Not only should you register everything they are saying and take mental notes, you must also be aware of what they are leaving out. (The British love of understatement, irony and sarcasm can trip you up if you are not careful here!)
- **Observe their body language:** Really look at how they are behaving as they are talking: their body language, gestures and facial expressions. This can give you an indication of how they feel about each topic and which ones you may want to ask them more about.

- **It's all about them:** Keep the focus on the other person. Continue to ask, *"How does that make you feel?"* and *"Please, tell me more about ..."* or even, *"What do you think you could do to change that?"* By throwing the ball back into their court and letting them talk, they may just solve their own problem.

PAUSE FOR THOUGHT

Vital Elements of Listening

- What are the main things that you will take away from this chapter?
- Which things have struck you most forcefully in this Step so far?

BODY LANGUAGE

As if you didn't have enough to think about, remember that your body language is hugely important. Your body is communicating with the speaker all the time you are silent and listening, and while the likelihood that they are aware of it consciously is slim to non-existent, they will certainly react instinctively.

- **Open-body stance:** Keeping your body open – not crossing your legs or arms – helps to show your interest, as does leaning slightly toward the speaker.
- **Eye contact:** Eye contact is an important way of showing that you are concentrating and not fiddling with your phone, watching TV or actively watching something else going on. However, you need to know when to make eye contact and when to avoid it. Many men find it easier not to make eye contact when they are spilling their soul, so my barber's position is ideal, partly because the listener has something to do and partly because they can use the subtle reflected glance in the mirror to good effect. You may be able to reproduce a similar position when seated in a car or on a park bench. Sometimes sitting next to each other is more impactful than sitting opposite and is much less confrontational.
- **Touch:** We must not underestimate the importance and power of human touch and physical connection. As a barber, I may be trimming a beard or running my fingers through their beard or hair – which is fairly intimate, especially between men. If appropriate, a hand on the shoulder or arm may make a huge difference, as it not only lets someone know you are listening to and empathizing with them, but it also releases the feel-good hormone oxytocin.

- **Personal space:** If you are close to the person – a partner or son, perhaps – then the rules change, as you may want to hug them or hold their hand. Whatever the physical connection, it should be appropriate for the relationship and for that particular moment. Consider that even your spouse might not want you to intrude on their own personal space when they are telling you something that is troubling them. Make sure you respect personal space and don't get so close that it makes them, or you, feel uncomfortable. The right approach will vary hugely between individuals, so you need to be alert to signals; for example, if they try to move away from you or cross their arms or legs to form a barrier.

- **Turn your head:** A subtle turn of the head toward the individual, just slightly showing them your ear, can actually be quite powerful and can encourage them to continue. Nodding your head in the right places is important, but you can't get away with just nodding and saying "Uh huh" without being fully engaged – that is not enough, and the speaker will spot it pretty easily.

- **Mirroring:** This actually happens naturally when people are communicating well, which makes it easier for you! If you watch a young couple talking, they will instinctively mirror each other's behaviour, both leaning in or touching each other's hair, and so on. If you do this consciously, it is better to partially mimic the speaker's behaviour, such as how they are sitting or resting their head on their chin, which can subconsciously let them know you are paying attention and are focused on them in the moment.

PAUSE FOR THOUGHT

Listening with Your Body

- Think back to an important conversation you've had. Reflect on your behaviour and how your body language may have influenced the conversation.
- If you were at levels 2 or 3, what would you do with your body language to bring that up to level 4? How would it impact the conversation?
- What would you do to bring that up to level 5?

CONTROLLING YOUR REACTIONS

When giving the Four-Step training, I am often asked: *"What if I don't like what I hear?"*

Unfortunately, at any stage of the process there will be things said that you may not like to hear, which is why we often avoid deep conversations or meaningful questions in the first place –

no one wants to hear that someone they know is struggling, especially if it is someone they love. It is distressing to hear and can be devastating. But *not* telling us their problems will only leave them struggling alone.

"Take a few deep breaths and stay calm. Don't let your reaction shock them back into silence now you have come this far."

If you have got past the fear of asking and have made it into the listening phase, then you have already done incredibly well. It's important to keep control when they tell you something that panics you, breaks your heart or even defines *you* as part of the problem.

Despite your heart sinking, your chest tightening and you beginning to sweat, take a few deep breaths and stay calm. Don't let your reaction shock them back into silence now you have come this far.

To demonstrate how important this is, think about your relationships – with your parents, for example. If they were the type of people who would shout and tell you off if you spilt something or came home late, would you tell them everything?

Would you talk to them about other stuff? Did they know what you were up to or who you were with? On the other hand, if your parents were the sort of people who helped you clean up or welcomed you home with a cup of tea and asked if you'd had a good night, would you have told them more as you knew there wouldn't be a negative reaction?

It's impossible to completely mask an instinctive reaction (just as you can't stop your leg kicking out if the doctor hits it below your kneecap), so you need to be prepared and do your best if someone you are talking to says something devastating. Don't ignore the emotion, but show it in a way that lets the other person know this is still a safe, non-judgemental environment. Try to refrain from jumping in and letting your emotions take over and start leading the conversation, which could result in feelings of sadness, anger, guilt or other emotions that we must try to curb at that point and for both parties; let the other person speak.

Try to keep your facial reaction neutral, but let them know you're still listening. Nod your head in agreement, and say simple things that let them know you are taking it on board and are comfortable to be told more. You might say:

- *"It must be really hard for you to tell me this."*
- *"I hear you."*
- *"I really appreciate you telling me."*

This also keeps them comfortable and allows them to say something that they probably never thought they would be able to tell you. When they have finished talking and realize what a safe space you are, it will mean so much more and will help build a strong bond – which is a very powerful thing.

Remember the importance of physical touch, and how (when used appropriately) it can make both of you feel better.

PAUSE FOR THOUGHT

Reactions

Think about your own reactions to hearing something shocking or upsetting. Are there some instinctive reactions that you would rather not share?

Think of some ways you might disguise them in the moment to encourage the speaker to continue to feel safe.

WHAT NOT TO SAY

When I look back at some of the things I have said to others, thinking I was helping them, or how I have reacted to someone's change in behaviour or low mood, I sometimes cringe; so don't worry if you do the same! Some of the guidance below will probably seem obvious, but it's important for us to cover it, as you may find some of these phrases creeping into your comments as you listen, without meaning to.

DON'T BE DISMISSIVE

It is important that we don't say anything that could be construed as dismissive. Such as:

- *"Cheer up mate, it can't be that bad."*
- *"Other people have problems too."*
- *"It could be worse!"*
- *"It's not the end of the world."*

Something that might initially seem unimportant to you may simply be the last straw or be a trigger – bringing with it deeper and more powerful issues.

DON'T BE AGGRESSIVE

If we are over-assertive, or even aggressive, the other person will feel attacked and is likely to shut down completely. Men especially are good at pretending to be OK and they are unlikely to confide in you if you put them on the defensive. So don't say:

- *"Don't be so grumpy."*
- *"It's not that big a deal!"*
- *"What's wrong with you?"*

DON'T COMPARE THEIR ISSUES WITH OTHERS

Avoid starting to talk about yourself or relate anecdotes about someone else; they will feel as though you have opened the door a crack then firmly closed it in their face.

- *"You should try ..."*
- *"You think you have it bad ..."*
- *"My friend had something similar ..."*

The only time this is useful is if someone feels like they are the only person who feels that way/or is going through that issue. In that situation, a brief mention of another's experience might be helpful.

DON'T LOOK AHEAD

If someone is in a difficult place, they are often immersed in it completely and can't see over the top of the hole they feel they are in, let alone see the horizon, so avoid clichés about the healing power of time, such as:

- *"It'll pass."*
- *"Time is a great healer."*
- *"Give it time."*

Concentrate on the now. There's plenty of time to discuss the future, but it's not helpful right now. They are probably not in a good-enough space to be able to take future possibilities on board.

PAUSE FOR THOUGHT

What Not to Say

As you read this section, you might be recalling a time when you said an unhelpful statement to someone. I am pretty sure we have all been there, and this might be the reason why you are reading this book.

Think of a time you have said something that you would now view as unhelpful … but don't dwell too long on it or beat yourself up over it. Instead, reflect on how you might handle the conversation in a different way now. What would you do differently, and how could you use that in the future?

RECOGNIZE, ASK, LISTEN, REPEAT

These Steps will keep repeating throughout your conversation as it progresses. You RECOGNIZE there is a change in behaviour, you build up the courage to ASK that person how they are really feeling and then you LISTEN.

As you listen, you may recognize something – they are having issues with money, for example – so maybe you ask them about that.

Then you listen further, and part of that listening will enable you to recognize that their money worries are because they are secretly gambling, so you can ask them about whether they feel as though they should speak to someone about it.

Then you listen some more until you reach some kind of resolution. It really is a continual process, and the more you do the more you will be able to see it working.

PROTECT YOURSELF

Please remember that if you feel distressed or hurt emotionally because of what you're told, then you need to offload and disclose how it made you feel. Have a think about who is in YOUR support network. There's more on this later in the book.

CONFIDENTIALITY

Confidentiality can be a tricky subject when it comes to dealing with people's mental wellbeing – especially suicidal thoughts and plans. It is also something that I have explored a fair bit when talking to other organizations in the UK like Samaritans, the UK National Suicide Prevention Helpline (called the National Suicide Prevention Lifeline in the USA) or mental health professionals and medical leads – and it always comes back to the same conclusion.

If the person who has disclosed their concerns to you is at immediate risk to themselves or others and you fear that it may end in someone losing their life or being hurt, you are allowed to report that to whoever may need to know, from a family member to the emergency services. It is best to make a plan with the individual first, but if that doesn't happen and you are still worried, then it is acceptable to tell others about the situation and the seriousness of it.

CONFIDENTIALITY IN PRACTICE

One morning, I picked up a message on the salon's Facebook page from a client – with whom I had discussed his poor mental health in many open conversations – saying that he was attempting suicide at that moment.

I immediately messaged him, and he told me where he was and that he was alone and in the process of taking his life. I managed to calm the rising panic and contact a mutual friend, and we called an ambulance. However, I did not know until that point that, in the UK, if you are conscious and somewhere private, you can refuse the help of the paramedics, which is what he did.

We continued to speak with him online to try to keep him alive, until he told us he was going for a walk. Since this took him into a public place, we were able to call the police, who were able to take him to safety. He is still alive today and is thankful that we were able to keep him alive.

LISTENING SKILLS

Once you have acquired your listening skills, you can apply them to every aspect of your life to good effect.

At home, you can be more aware of the subtext of conversations, and get more in tune with your family or housemates.

At work, you will be in a good position to really understand what the boss is asking for or what colleagues are telling you.

In social situations, you'll become known as a good listener and will be able to support your friends in the most useful ways.

When there's a problem, you'll be the one they come to when they need to get something off their chest.

PAUSE FOR THOUGHT

Check Your Confidence Scores

Go back to page 27 and run through the confidence questions again.

How do you score now?

LISTENING DOS AND DON'TS

- Don't interrupt.
- Don't tell them you know how they feel.
- Don't fill silences.
- Don't try to "fix" or "solve" anything.
- Do reassure them you're listening, either by mimicking, body language, or repeating their words, or encouraging them to tell you more about it.
- Do tell them that you want to them to explain their feelings to you.
- Do give them time to speak – silences are often because they are trying to work out how to say what they are thinking.
- Do have knowledge of resources and professionals you can direct them to.

6

STEP FOUR: HELP

The final Step is HELP: guiding people toward whatever services or support they need to restore their mental health. To start, I would like you to write down all the services you already know of that you could signpost someone to or seek help from yourself.

PAUSE FOR THOUGHT

Sources of Support

How many services do you know about that help people with mental health issues?

Give yourself a couple of minutes. See if you can think of more than five.

I am assuming that with all the current campaigning and recognition of mental health, combined with the fact that you bought this book, you may have a few ideas. That's great!

Unfortunately, a lot of people I ask can't name *any*. And neither could I, until my friend Alex ended his life. We all know where look for help with our physical health, yet when it comes to mental health, we have a lot to learn. In this part of the book, I hope to help you change that.

The first three phases – RECOGNIZE, ASK, LISTEN – may, in fact, be enough to help the individual. Allowing them to talk through their issues may bring them to their own solutions, and can be enormously cathartic in itself.

Some of those we talk with may be clinically depressed or have other diagnosed mental conditions, but many will simply want to talk about the ups and downs of everyday life and let off steam about work, relationships, bereavement, money issues, parenting – all things that can affect our mental wellbeing. Sometimes a listening ear is all that is needed to encourage people to help themselves.

GETTING SUPPORT YOURSELF

I have often found that after teaching a BarberTalk course, the people taking the course have recognized things within themselves that they would like to offload about or seek further support with. We should never forget that you cannot pour from an empty cup – we all need support sometimes.

So, before we move on to how we can help, I want to point out that if you find that you are the one who is struggling, or it is becoming difficult to support those around you, please remember that you can access and use anything that is mentioned in this chapter.

It is important to remember this, because even though you are most likely to be a supporter and see yourself as a helper of others, at times you will need help too.

GUIDING PEOPLE TO THE RIGHT SUPPORT

As you're not a medical practitioner or mental health expert, this stage can feel a bit unnerving (although maybe you have felt like this before reading other chapters too!).

The great thing is, however, you don't need to be a mental health professional to be able to help someone; and the even better news is that there is an abundance of resources out there that are available to those struggling.

When I am facilitating this Step during a live training session, we have a simple exercise where I separate the group into smaller teams and ask them to "warm up their search engines": to conduct an online search for what resources are available in their area. They are often happily surprised at how much is actually available to those in need.

Because services and facilities are often localized, it is much better to undertake your own research, although the Useful Resources section on page 171 contains some to get you started. Remember that you are looking for support that is specific to the person in question, so not all recommendations are going to be suitable for everyone. You will need to pick and choose.

BASIC HELPLINES AND FIRST STEPS

A good starting point is to pass on to the person you are talking with their local or national mental health helpline, to make sure they are aware of them and have the right contact details.

Many countries, including the USA, UK, Canada and Australia, have national helplines available 24/7. There are also some fantastic charities offering support and help. See the Useful

Resources chapter for the details of these, and text the information to the person you're helping. It's a good first step.

It may also be appropriate to encourage the person that you are supporting to seek medical help from their doctor (see page 134).

In severe cases, when you have no idea what to do in the moment, the emergency services – ambulance and police – are available to help. There are also usually mental health professionals and crisis teams at the accident and emergency rooms.

CHOOSING THE RIGHT MEDIUM

How you decide what is right to suggest to the person looking for help is a matter of narrowing down the options. Think about all the different ways in which we can communicate and gather information today; it is greater than it has ever been.

Consider whether you think the person you are supporting would benefit from reading a self-help book, connecting with likeminded people on social media, using a counselling texting or video call service, face-to-face meetings, an exercise activity, or group or individual therapy.

There are so many ways to connect and support one another. If you are unsure as to what would best suit your person in need, ask them what they would prefer and go down that route to search for resources that may fit their preferences.

LOCAL RESOURCES

Once you have confirmed the kind of help you think the person would respond to, start researching what is available in your area.

> "The great thing is, you don't need to be a mental health professional to be able to help someone ... there is an abundance of resources out there."

Check out local groups, which are often run by those who have experienced poor mental health themselves or within their social circle. They are always very welcoming and passionate about the cause.

A great example of this kind of resource is the fantastic Dudes and Dogs group in Bristol, southwest England, which involves a few guys regularly meeting up, with their dogs, and going for a walk. There's also an organization in the UK called Andy's Man Club, which organizes regular social get-togethers for men.

Men are often far better at talking while doing, which is why you find similar groups that revolve around mechanics, football, gardening or fitness. These peer support groups seem to be particularly attractive to men, as well as being far more effective.

Ask the person you are supporting if it's OK for you to share with them some of the organizations you've found. They will need to take the necessary action to become involved, but you can always offer to go along with them to an event. Many online helplines can be anonymous, which may encourage them to reach out.

PAUSE FOR THOUGHT

Resources to Recommend

Make a list of all the resources that you think might help someone – both national helplines and small local groups. Keep this list somewhere safe, and add to it if you discover other organizations that might be helpful.

This will be your "Keepsafe Connections", and it should be updated regularly to ensure the services are still operating.

It never hurts to recommend a group or resource to someone. It doesn't mean they have to act on it, but it might just be the nudge they need.

THE BEST WAYS TO HELP MEN

Research by the UK charity Samaritans aimed to understand how to engage men earlier and thus avoid their mental health issues becoming so serious they result in suicide attempts. They did this by speaking with men across the UK and Ireland through workshops, and explored what activities and initiatives could support their wellbeing and hopefully prevent them reaching a crisis point.

They found that the men preferred wellbeing-led activities over clinical mental health or crisis services, and gravitated toward hobby-based groups or activities; they appreciated that such groups and activities developed friendships through shared interests, often in traditional "male" activities like sport.

For me, the most important outcome of the research is the fact that Samaritans concluded that there was no "one-size-fits-all" solution to the problem, which I heartily agree with. This can be difficult, though, as it means it's worth knowing as many different options as possible, as you never know when they will come in useful.

SEEING THE DOCTOR

One of the obvious ways for many to find help would be to make an appointment to see their doctor.

The Lions Barber Collective conducted a survey with shaving products company Bluebeards Revenge in 2018, which confirmed that most men see their barber more than they see their doctor, and they would also rather talk to their barber than their doctor about their mental health!

I imagine the men in your life have had their hair cut, beard trimmed or shaved more times this year than seeing their doctor. We need to change the stigma around going to the doctor, so do think of them as a possible first port of call, if the sufferer agrees.

MEDICATION

Taking medication for depression or other similar conditions is not a magic treatment – it won't be appropriate for some people and there can be difficult side effects. That said, it can be life-changing for many. When someone is depressed, they have an imbalance of chemicals in the brain, which is what the medication is designed to address. The medication does not solve the problem, but it can help the person to regain control sufficiently to begin the healing process themselves. It can help someone emerge from the dark place they were in, and free up energy to restore their mental health. Again, seeing your doctor is the right first step down this path.

The doctor may recommend medication or make a referral to other mental health services, which may be able to diagnose the situation and start the recovery process. This can be combined with other group activities, therapy or peer support, which together can have a positive outcome.

Often there's a waiting period for mental health services, which is why it's so important for you to keep in touch and keep having conversations while they may be waiting for additional help.

HELPING THEM HELP THEMSELVES

It is worth recapping your role in helping them help themselves.

Your role is to remain calm and reassuring, to listen and to suggest. You are not looking to make their problems disappear, or tell them how you feel or what your own answers would be, or offer them ready-made solutions.

By listening to their assessment of the situation, you might realize that they are actually suggesting what they think they should do, or would like to do, and you can reinforce that and then create a plan with them to take whatever action is appropriate.

This is where active listening to so powerful.

HOW YOU CAN CONTINUE TO HELP

There are plenty of things you can do to help the ones we love on an ongoing basis.

CONVERSATIONS

Encouraging conversations is vital, and once we have had the initial, most difficult conversation, this should become a bit easier each time you communicate.

Check in on how they received the resource that you suggested. Did they follow it up? Is the support service helpful? Also, show your interest in their recovery and let them know they can continue to talk to you.

> "Being there for someone – to sit with them, hold them and reassure them – can go an awfully long way, much further than telling them what to do or trying to fix an issue for them."

KEEPING IN TOUCH

If you can, then continuing to check in with them regularly is probably the simplest form of help – and possibly the most valuable – because that person knows that you continue to care for them, value them and want them to be around.

We all need to belong and to love and be loved (it is a vital human requirement), and being there for someone – to sit with them, hold them and reassure them – can go an awfully long way, much further than telling them what to do or trying to fix an issue for them. If you're struggling to find the time or mental capacity to do this, try encouraging another of their loved ones to make contact. You don't need to tell them the real reason – you could just say that your mutual friend would appreciate a message.

PASSING ON THE TASK

It can be a very difficult thing to do when we care so much, but you may not be the right person to provide the necessary support, and that takes a big person to realize. There may well be better people for that role, and by getting those people on side and adding to the sufferer's support group may be better for both you and the sufferer.

Have a think about who is in your/their family group or close social circle who may be a better listener or offer a different kind of practical support, if you feel uncomfortable in this role.

Crucially, this does not make you a failure. In fact, it's the complete opposite – that decision could save a life!

OTHER WAYS OF HELPING

If this book leads you to start a worthy conversation with just one person, then this will all have been worth it. You may also decide to store your knowledge of the Steps and be vigilant for signs among those closest to you – that's brilliant.

Below are some ideas about how you can help the mental health conversation further grow and develop, in addition to having those conversations.

BUDDY UP

You could implement a "buddying up" process at your place of work, where each of you has a buddy and you check in on each other daily, just to ask, "How are you feeling today?", and keep up to date on each other's day-to-day life.

This is simple but effective, and has been used to great success in some high-pressure environments, like the Nightingale Hospitals (during the Covid-19 pandemic in the UK), where a mental health focus was implemented to ensure the wellbeing of those on site before they started their shift. Having that individual support can be a game-changer.

VOLUNTEER

If you have a bit more drive – and the time, too – you could potentially volunteer for one of the many charities or organizations that are already doing a great job in your area or nationally.

Charities and non-profits are always keen to have volunteers, and I can honestly say that if it wasn't for the volunteers who help with the Lions Barber Collective, we simply wouldn't be the charity we are today; they are essential to the success of what we do and have saved lives, without a doubt.

You may have found some organizations during your research that hit home with you; you could offer some of your time to keep them successfully helping others.

GO IT ALONE

This book is primarily aimed at starting simple, everyday conversations about mental health. That said, if you have the time, energy and passion, setting up your own support group or charity could be an amazing thing. Don't underestimate how all-consuming it can be – and I'm talking from experience! – but it is also hugely rewarding.

If you do decide to go down this route, go for something that offers an activity that is not already available locally. This could be a walking group for men in your area, a gardening collective working a plot of land together, an open-water swimming group, regular get-togethers based around a quiz or sport, group counselling services, or anything else you can come up with and that you have experience of.

If this is something that you want to pursue, please take a look at local rules and regulations and contact your local council and public health, as they would probably be keen to help you in some way and have all the information you need to make your project a success.

PAUSE FOR THOUGHT

How Confident Are You Now?

Before you move on, take a penultimate look at the confidence activity on page 27 once more. How confident do you feel now?

7

WHAT IF THE CONVERSATION GOES WRONG?

In my experience, an attempt to begin a genuine conversation is always well received. It may not always have gone the way I expected – maybe it wasn't quite the right time, or maybe I misread the situation slightly – but people have always been grateful and warm toward the opportunity to have a proper chat.

It may be that you plan everything perfectly, but the conversation doesn't progress how you expected. You can pick the right time, the right place and ask all the right questions, but that person may not want to talk at that moment or you may get interrupted.

If that happens, don't worry. Don't get frustrated or try to continue the conversation if the situation or timing is no longer right – simply endeavour to have that conversation again soon.

If you feel the situation is particularly serious and the conversation needs to be had urgently, then reach out and make it a priority:

"I feel like we got interrupted then! What are you doing later? Do you want to go for a walk and finish what we were saying?"

WHAT IF THEY SHUT YOU DOWN?

Many people have asked this question when I have been facilitating the BarberTalk course, and it is a valid one.

If the person says they are OK – even if you're fairly convinced that they aren't – that can feel very final and end that opportunity instantly. To avoid an awkward pause before you move on or part ways, have your response ready. In this situation I would always apologise briefly and reply with a simple but effective answer:

"Sorry. I'm glad you're OK. I only asked because I care about you, but I'm here if you do ever want to talk."

That can make many people pause. You'll almost see them think it over in their head, and sometimes they'll come back with:

"Actually, there is something …"

It can be as easy as that; they just needed to be given another opportunity to feel safe.

If they don't come back to you straightaway, then you have at least let them know that you can provide a safe space to speak. That is half the battle.

It's worth bearing in mind that the person you're worried about may genuinely be absolutely fine, and you had no reason to worry!

"You've shown you care, which is a big thing."

Your first enquiring question is likely to be fairly innocuous, so if the answer you get convinces you that the guy is actually OK, move on in a different direction with something more trivial, like the weather, the football or their plans. Sometimes we'll misread signals – that can happen no matter how refined your observation skills! Again, you've shown you care, which is a big thing.

If (and this is unlikely) the person reacts badly to your attempt to start a conversation, the most important thing is not to take it personally. If the person is offended by your question, be sensitive. Give a brief apology, diffuse any negative feelings, and let them know that you were worried because you care – then get back to the weather!

I cannot imagine anyone being that upset about you genuinely caring about their wellbeing. It may be that you have hit the nail on the head, but they are not ready to open up.

> "The important thing is not to push it. If someone isn't ready to open up, then pushing them could do more harm than good."

Perhaps you could generalize the conversation and tell them about a charity such as the Lions Barbers Collective with no reference to them, giving them enough information so that they know where to go when they are ready.

Or simply just let them know, if they should want to speak to you, you are there. The important thing, though, is not to push it. If someone isn't ready to open up in that moment, then pushing them could do more harm than good.

You have probably heard the expression, "You can lead a horse to water, but you can't make it drink". This is, unfortunately, often the case. You cannot make someone talk; you can only encourage them and let them know that they can come to you in future. This may sound final and difficult, and it is. The hope is by letting them know you are a safe, non-judgemental person then they will feel comfortable and confident enough to confide in you at some point.

PERMISSION TO SPEAK

There are lots of occasions now where I don't even have to ask. I can be out for an evening and someone will recognize me and proceed to offload to me about their mental health or a situation that is affecting their mental health.

I have been publicly telling people it is OK to talk to me for five years, so that's on me!

I am not asking you to become a public agony aunt or uncle, but by letting a person know that they can message you or email you, call you or even just come up to you tomorrow at work, you have done something incredible!

8

BUILDING BLOCKS TO POSITIVE MENTAL HEALTH

I hope you feel that you now are better equipped to help those around you from learning how to RECOGNIZE, ASK, LISTEN and HELP. It's also crucial that while doing this, you also to keep an eye on your own mental health.

This chapter aims to help you recognize mental health areas that could be improved. It will look at the basics of keeping our minds healthy, so we can maintain our own mental strength. The British National Health Service suggests several simple building blocks to help you achieve and maintain mental wellbeing. I have taken these as a starting point and expanded on them.

PAUSE FOR THOUGHT

How Might These Building Blocks Help the Person You Want to Help?

While reading this chapter, consider whether you could suggest any lifestyle changes to the man you want to help. This will obviously depend on your relationship with him, and whether it's an appropriate topic to discuss, but bringing up a subject such as "How are you sleeping?" could open up a conversation about this, and may lead to some positive changes.

This section also equally applies to you. If you have been affected by the stress of trying to care for someone with mental health problems, it will be particularly important to find ways to deal with that stress and minimize its negative effects. Following some of the ideas in this chapter should help. Remember, you can't pour from an empty cup!

No two readers will need to do the same things to maintain their mental health, because we are all different and have different routines and lifestyles. I'm not going to tell you what you must or must not do.

PAUSE FOR THOUGHT

Create Your Own Mental Health "Manual"

Look at each building block in this chapter, and think about what it means in terms of your life, because everyone's ways of implementing these elements will be different. You may be surprised to find that you are already doing several of these blocks which is great.

Then, map out a few easy things that you can do to help ensure that you are engaging with each block. You should then have a plan for moving forward and looking after your own mental fitness.

CONNECT WITH OTHERS

All human beings need to love, be loved and to have a sense of belonging. The opposite – isolation and loneliness – play a huge role in mental ill health. Connection with others will not only enable you to feel as though you belong to something, but also feed your feelings of self-worth. That's kind of why I want to encourage conversation, funnily enough!

Most of us can relate to feeling part of a team, and how good that feels. In those moments when everyone is working together, we can share stories, create positive memories and develop the bonds between us. At the same time, we may also share some not-so-positive experiences – but working together to find solutions together serves to bind us even further. These teams or groups can also provide support for you when you need it most.

There are of course numerous online groups you can join, but, in my opinion, there is no substitute for real human contact and conversation. There are options for everyone: meeting someone for coffee, going for a walk, team sports, crafts … the list is endless. Consider finding a group for a hobby you enjoy and going along with a friend. It can be scary, but these groups often have a real sense of community.

Connecting with others also crucial for your wellbeing, as it strengthens your support network. Think of it as one large chain – we each need people who we can to talk to and who can support us, just as we support others. For you to help others, it's vital you have people you can turn to.

PHYSICAL ACTIVITY

Regular exercise can have a huge positive effect on mental health, especially in helping to lift depression and dispel anxiety, relieve excess stress, improve sleep and boost your mood.

Combine this chemical rush with the known benefits of fresh air and nature, and outdoor exercise becomes a powerful building block to positive mental health. Getting out in the fresh air to exercise in nature has huge benefits mentally. Exercise also provides a rush of positive chemical changes in your brain. Most people understand that endorphins are released when we exercise, but the brain also releases the feel-good, mood-regulating dopamine, norepinephrine and serotonin, all of which means that our physical activity is important to mental fitness.

DIET

All this physical activity needs the right fuel, too, so make sure you're not neglecting your diet. Your diet can drastically affect both your physical and mental health in a range of ways. Speak to your doctor to make sure your diet is right for you – and that you're drinking enough water!

Physical exercise may also prove to be the perfect way to engage the person you're worried about. A run or a walk can be a great opportunity for a chat – this exercise could be your route to an important conversation. You can think outside the box here: maybe suggest something new you could try together, such as paddleboarding.

GET SOME SLEEP

Rest and sleep are also important to let your body and your mind wind down after the exertions of the day. If you have trouble sleeping, there are plenty of things you can do to help you drift off.

- Remove technology from the bedroom – no laptops, iPads or games consoles.
- Have a bedtime slow-down routine.
- Think about the temperature of your room – be warm but not hot, cool but not cold.
- Never underestimate the value of a comfortable, good-quality mattress and pillow.
- Try to avoid heavy alcoholic drinking.
- Have a break between your last meal of the day and bedtime.
- If you have worries or concerns stopping you from drifting off, write them down to get them out of your brain, or write down all the positive things you have done or achieved.

- Listen to soothing music, sleep stories or guided meditation.
- Read a book.
- Sometimes a power nap during the day will help you feel less tired and prevent you from being anxious and over-tired when you go to bed.

NEVER STOP LEARNING

Whenever I meet someone successful, I always ask if they have any advice, and the answer more often than not is, *"Never stop learning"*. So there has to be something in it, surely?

Learning new skills helps boost confidence and self-esteem. There's nothing like achievement to help with those two emotions. Your achievements don't have to be getting a PhD or learning to speak Mandarin – although they could be! They can be as simple as learning to cook your favourite meal or learning how to edit all those videos you take on your phone. It is about discovering what YOU want to learn more about and then doing it.

> "Learning new skills helps boost confidence and self-esteem. There's nothing like achievement to help with those two emotions."

This is a great block to gently encourage someone to build. Ask them what parts of their life they want to expand on – perhaps they have a rusty motorbike in the garage that they've been meaning to do up for years (or, like my friend Steve, a flat they can convert into a studio!)

GIVE AND BE KIND

Who'd have thought it – being kind reduces stress and makes everyone feel good. How simple is that?

I would say this is one of the biggest and easiest steps to take. A simple "hello" or "good morning" with a smile to someone you pass on the street can change their day!

I have a reminder set on my phone for 9:27am every Monday that simply says, "Text someone". It gives me a moment to pause and think about people who I have seen achieve something great over the past week, or someone I love or someone that I haven't spoken to in a while and send them a text. It may be one person, it could be several. But what better way to start the week than with a random text of support or love and, believe me, the responses are also a great way to start your week too.

"Acts of kindness give a sense of self-worth and positive feelings, as well as purpose and connection with others."

There are plenty of things you could do, like volunteering work, mentoring someone, sending an unexpected gift (just because), pay-forward a cup of coffee with your morning latte, or simply give up your seat on the train. All these things give a sense of self-worth and positive feelings, as well as purpose and connection with others.

START WITH A GIFT

In Thailand, Buddhists believe that the first thing they do every morning should be a kind thing, so they might make someone a cup of tea, feed the birds or even just smile at a stranger.

BE PRESENT IN THE MOMENT

Sometimes referred to as mindfulness, being in the moment is hugely important to wellbeing. Mindfulness is paying attention to every detail of what is happening to you now, and not worrying about a past that can't be changed or a future that can't be controlled. We spend a lot of our time distracted and worrying about these things, which can spiral out of control internally. There are so many things fighting for our attention that we become unable to concentrate on anything, and have to react to each stimulus as it beeps into our consciousness.

Being in the moment can be whatever we want it to be as long as we are focusing on that and that alone. The first thing I try to remember is: control the controllable. We can only control our own thoughts and actions, so try not to fret about things outside of that and be present in your thoughts and actions. Focus instead on all your senses and what they are telling you right now.

HOW TO BE IN THE MOMENT (MY VERSION)

True mindfulness is achieved through meditation, which many of you may have tried with a greater or lesser degree of success. We all have our own perceptions of what "being in the moment" involves, and might feel a little daunted by it.

If you're a novice, I would actually recommend you don't begin by trying out a meditation exercise! Instead, here are some starter ideas for how to stay in the moment. They may not be what you'd normally associate with mindfulness, so hopefully they'll encourage you to think out of the box a little, and beyond meditation.

- **Listen to music through headphones:** Choose some of your favourite tracks, close your eyes and concentrate on the music.
- **Eat mindfully:** Notice each bite you take, with no distractions. Notice the textures and tastes.
- **Take a walk outside:** Observe nature all around you, listen to the birdsong and smell that fresh air. Really focus on your different senses.
- **Count the clouds:** Lie on your back in the sun and look for shapes in the clouds as they move above you.
- **Go to the cinema:** A darkened room, no interruptions and a great film – what's not to like? Unlike TV at home, your phone won't be going off, people won't be coming to the door and children won't be screaming for your attention.
- **Go for a haircut or a professional wet shave:** Well, I would say that, wouldn't I?

The importance of doing day-to-day things more mindfully can make a huge difference to your wellbeing. That peace and pause in your hectic lifestyle is crucial and, in essence, that's mindfulness.

CONTROL THE CONTROLLABLE

One of the reasons it is so important for your mental health to not to spend too much time in the past or the future is that those places are outside of your control. The only things we have control over are our thoughts and our actions – that's it!

And before you start thinking that's a bit unnerving, look at it another way: it is also extremely liberating. Let's say someone is unkind to us – that's not our fault and there's nothing we could have done to stop it. The only choices we have is how we deal with it. We can choose to dwell on it and let it continue to make us unhappy, or we can let it go.

"You can only provide a safe space, ask the right questions, and their response is beyond your control."

Earlier in the book we spoke about a conversation not going the way we planned. If that happens, it's crucial to remember that you did all you could in that moment, and you can't control how someone else reacts. You can only provide a safe space, ask the right questions – their response is beyond your control. We can continue to learn and continue to support people, but we can't force them to react the way we want them to.

You should also set personal boundaries, which will help you protect your own mental health. If you need time to recharge and recover from your interactions with the man who is struggling, then take it. You can always ask a mutual friend to reach out to the man you're trying to help, or encourage that man to talk to one of the many services available. It's vital that you protect yourself, otherwise you won't be able to help anyone. As well as being beneficial to the man in question, signposting them to other resources also means you're not shouldering that huge emotional weight alone.

MAKING SMALL CHANGES

My hope is that this brief chapter on mental wellbeing may flag some areas for you to work on,

It's so important to start small – even tiny changes to your life can hugely affect your mental wellbeing. Step outside the front door, or stick your head out the window first thing in the morning for a breath of fresh air. That's just 10 seconds out of your day!

I also hope this chapter may lead you to make gentle suggestions to someone you see as struggling with their mental health. Could you suggest a new hobby (learning opportunity) you think they might enjoy? Could you invite them out for a walk (ticking off both physical and mindful activities)? Could you suggest a local group that would foster connection and maybe some physical exercise?

Remember, through the very act of trying to have the conversation, trying to actively listen, you will be giving someone the opportunity for further connection – with you.

FINAL THOUGHTS: YOU CAN MAKE A DIFFERENCE

In this book, we have covered a range of skills that will help you to begin conversations and actively listen to friends, loved ones, colleagues or even strangers about their mental health. We have specifically focused on talking to men about their mental health, acknowledging that men's mental health is a complex subject where our gentle questions and active listening can make a real difference.

"If you are prepared to hold out a helping hand to a man who needs it, you will make a difference."

We have gone through the Four-Step process of

- RECOGNIZING that a problem may exist,
- building up the courage to ASK pertinent questions,

- LISTENING with patience and without judgement,
- and have developed our knowledge of resources that are out there to support and HELP anyone who is troubled by mental health issues, whether mild or serious.

We've looked at how a conversation may not go as planned, and what can be done in the most serious of situations. We have also considered how we can maintain our own good mental health, and how to encourage others do the same.

No one is suggesting any of this will be easy but that doesn't mean we shouldn't try.

If you are prepared to hold out a helping hand to a man who needs it, you will make a difference. Whether that is simply cheering their mood or letting them talk through and resolve a decision, or guiding them to professional help for a serious mental health issue, all our equally valuable for the recipient of your support. At its most extreme, your support could be saving a life.

PAUSE FOR THOUGHT

Measure Your Confidence

Right at the beginning of the book, you answered a series of questions about your confidence in your own ability to help and support others (page 27). Now you have read the whole book, look at those questions again.

Compare the two sets of results. Hopefully you will have grown both in confidence and knowledge, and feel ready to listen in a way that will make a male in your life open up and talk to you.

So, ask that opening question.

Be aware of opportunities and use them.

Be observant of men's behaviour and have the courage to offer a gesture of support.

Learn to communicate at an emotional level.

Learn to truly listen.

If we can do those things, we will all benefit.

Together we can make a difference – a huge difference.

Thank you for reading this book and caring about others. Care for them, and make sure you care for yourself too.

ACKNOWLEDGEMENTS

Thank you to my boys, Abel and Drake, for whom I hope that my efforts now may make a difference to their mental wellbeing when they grow up to be men.

Thanks go to Dr Peter Aitken, for seeing value in all of my dreams and wild ideas, and supporting them and me throughout the journey so far. And to Gini Holden, for believing in me and empowering me to turn ideas into realities to support not only others but also me and my family.

Thank you Wendy Hobson, Matt Tomlinson and Beth Bishop for their work on this book. Thanks also to Dale at One Tribe Talent for believing in me.

Thank you to my parents, for always making me feel safe, and for teaching me that failure was a means to success, while inspiring me and teaching me about work ethic and entrepreneurism.

Finally, thank you to the woman who has enabled me to do everything and achieve more than I could have imagined:

my wife, Tenneille. She has supported my travel to the other ends of the globe for work and has forgiven the extra hours I have given to both the charity, my training model, hair and my dreams. I wouldn't be half the man I am without her in my life.

REFERENCES

Chapter 1

Australian Institute of Health and Welfare. 'Suicide & self-harm monitoring'. [Online] Available at: www.aihw.gov.au/suicide-self-harm-monitoring [Accessed 19 November 2021].

Office for National Statistics. 'Suicides in England and Wales'. [Online] Available at: www.ons.gov.uk/peoplepopulationand community/birthsdeathsandmarriages/deaths/bulletins/suicides intheunitedkingdom/2020registrations [Accessed 19 November 2021].

Public Health Scotland. 'Suicide prevention overview'. [Online] Available at: www.healthscotland.scot/health-topics/suicide/suicide-prevention-overview [Accessed 19 November 2021].

Northern Ireland Statistics and Research Agency. 'Suicide Deaths'. [Online] Available at: www.nisra.gov.uk/statistics/cause-death/suicide-deaths [Accessed 19 November 2021].

National Institute of Mental Health (NIMH). 'Suicide'. [Online] Available at: www.nimh.nih.gov/health/statistics/suicide [Accessed 19 November 2021].

Mental Health Foundation. 'Mental health statistics: men and women'. [Online]. Available at: www.mentalhealth.org.uk/ statistics/mental-health-statistics-men-and-women [Accessed 21 Oct. 2021]

Statista. 'Percentage of U.S. adults with any mental illness in the past year as of 2019, by age and gender'. [Online] Available at: www.statista.com/statistics/252311/mental-illness-in-the-past-year-among-us-adults-by-age-and-gender [Accessed 21 Oct. 2021]

Rice-Oxley, M. (2019). 'Why do so many construction workers kill themselves?' [online] Available at: www.theguardian.com/ society/2019/aug/13/why-do-so-many-construction-workers-kill-themselves [Accessed 21 Oct. 2021]

Brown, B. (2015). *Daring Greatly*. London: Avery Publishing Group.

The University of Manchester. 'Suicide by middle-aged men'. [Online]. Available at: documents.manchester.ac.uk/display. aspx?DocID=55305 [Accessed 19 November 2021].

National Institute of Mental Health (NIMH). 2021. 'Mental Illness'. [Online] Available at: www.nimh.nih.gov/health/statistics/mental-illness [Accessed 19 November 2021].

The University of Manchester. 'NCISH Annual Report (2008-2018)'. [Online] Available at: documents.manchester.ac.uk/display.aspx?DocID=55333 [Accessed 19 November 2021].

The Independent. 2021. Women are twice as likely as men to self-harm. *The Independent.* [Online] Available at: www.independent.co.uk/life-style/self-harm-young-adults-women-anxiety-eating-disorders-addiction-a8569811.html [Accessed 11 November 2021].

Priory. 2021. 'Supporting Men with Mental Health Issues'. [Online] Available at: www.priorygroup.com/blog/supporting-men-with-mental-health-issues [Accessed 19 November 2021].

SAVE. 2021. Suicide Statistics and Facts – SAVE. [Online] Available at: save.org/about-suicide/suicide-facts [Accessed 11 November 2021].

Chapter 4
IASP. IASP Home. [Online] Available at: www.iasp.info/suicide_and_the_media_members.php [Accessed 11 November 2021].

Owens, C. and Charles, N. (2017). 'Development and evaluation of a leaflet for concerned family members and friends: "It's safe to talk about suicide."' *Health Education Journal*, 76(5), pp.582–594.

Chapter 5
Medical News Today. 'Oxytocin: The love hormone?' [Online] Available at: www.medicalnewstoday.com/articles/275795 [Accessed 11 November 2021].

Chapter 6
Samaritans. 'Research into our services'. [Online] Available at: www.samaritans.org/about-samaritans/research-policy/research-our-services [Accessed 19 November 2021].

USEFUL RESOURCES

NATIONAL TEXT HELPLINES
www.crisistextline.org

CANADA & USA
Text 741741

UK & NORTHERN IRELAND
Text 85258

IRELAND
Text 50808

NATIONAL TELEPHONE HELPLINES
Australia
Emergency services: 000
Lifeline: 13 11 14

Canada
Canada Suicide Prevention Helpline: 1-833-456-4560
(NB: from 2023 it will be 988)
Emergency services: 911

New Zealand
Emergency services: 111
Need to talk: 1737

South Africa
Emergency services: 111 or 117
Suicide Crisis Line: 0800 567 657

UK and Ireland
Childline: 0800 1111
Emergency services: 999
Samaritans: 116 123

USA
Emergency services: 911
National Suicide Prevention Lifeline: 1-800-273-8255 (NB: from 2022, it will be 988)

SUICIDE PREVENTION ORGANIZATIONS
Australia
Lifeline Australia: lifeline.org.au
Suicide Prevention Australia (SPA): suicidepreventionaust.org

Canada
Canadian Association for Suicide Prevention (CASP):
suicideprevention.ca
Canada Suicide Prevention Crisis Service: crisisservicescanada.ca

International
Wikipedia: Wikipedia.org/List_of_suicide_crisis_lines

New Zealand
Supporting People in New Zealand (SPINZ): spinz.org.nz

South Africa
Lifeline South Africa: lifeline.org.sa

UK
Campaign Against Living Miserably (CALM): thecalmzone.net
Centre for Suicide Prevention: manchester.ac.uk (and search
suicide prevention)
Lions Barber Collective: lionsbarbercollective.com
PAPYRUS (prevention of young suicide): papyrus-uk.org

Samaritans: samaritans.org; Helpline: 116 123

SANE: sane.org.uk

Support After Suicide Partnership (UK): supportaftersuicide.org.uk

Survivors of Bereavement by Suicide (UK): uksobs.org

USA

Alliance of Hope (for suicide loss survivors): allianceofhope.org

American Association of Suicidology: suicidology.org

American Foundation for Suicide Prevention: afsp.org

International Association for Suicide Prevention (IASP): iasp.info

Jed Foundation (dedicated to the prevention of young suicide): *jedfoundation.org*

National Suicide Prevention Lifeline: suicidepreventionlifeline.org

GENERAL MENTAL HEALTH RESOURCES
Australia and New Zealand

Beyond Blue: beyondblue.org.au

Head to Health: headtohealth.gov.au

Health Direct: healthdirect.gov.au

Mental Health Australia: mhaustralia.org

Mental Health Foundation of New Zealand: mentalhealth.org.nz

SANE Australia: www.sane.org

Canada

Canadian Mental Health Association: cmha.ca

Crisis Service Canada: ementalhealth.ca

Europe

Mental Health Europe: mhe-sme.org

Mental Health Ireland: mentalhealthireland.ie

International

Therapy Route: therapyroute.com

UK

Diversity Trust: diversitytrust.org

Heads Together: headstogether.org.uk

Hub of Hope: hubofhope.co.uk

Mental Health Foundation UK: mentalhealth.org.uk

Mind UK: mind.org.uk

My Pickle: mypickle.org

NHS Mental Health: nhs.uk/mental-health

Rethink Mental Illness: rethink.org

Samaritans: samaritans.org, helpline: 116 123

Scottish Association for Mental Health (SAMH) (Scotland): samh.org.uk

Shout: giveusashout.org, text 85258

Young Minds: youngminds.org.uk

USA

Mentalhealth.gov: mentalhealth.gov

Mental Health America: mhanational.org

National Alliance on Mental Illness: nami.org

National Institute of Mental Health: nimh.nih.gov

Other countries

It's OK to Talk (India): itsoktotalk.in

Pan American Mental Health Organization (North and South America): www.paho.org

SPECIFIC ISSUES SUPPORT AND INFORMATION
Autism

National Autistic Society (UK): www.autism.org.uk

Autism Society (USA): www.autism-society.org

Autism Awareness (Australia): www.autismawareness.com.au

Bullying

Bullying UK: bullying.co.uk

Stomp Out Bullying (USA): stompoutbullying.org

Bully Zero (Australia): bullyzero.org.au

Carers

Carers UK: carersuk.org

Family Carers Ireland: familycarers.ie

National Alliance for Caregiving (USA): caregiving.org

Carers Canada: carerscanada.ca

Carers Australia: carersaustralia.com.au

Carers New Zealand: carers.net.nz

LGBTQ+

LBGT Foundation (UK): lgbt.foundation

Trevor Project (USA): thetrevorproject.org

Q Life counseling service (Australia): qlife.org.au

Psychological Societies and Associations

American Psychological Association: apa.org

Australian Psychological Society: psychology.org.au

British Psychological Society (UK): bps.org.uk

Canadian Psychological Association: cpa.org

Royal College of Psychiatrists (UK): rcpsych.ac.uk

ABOUT THE LIONS BARBER COLLECTIVE

The Lions Barber Collective is an international collective of top barbers, who have come together to help raise awareness for the prevention of suicide.

Run by volunteers, the charity attends industry shows and festivals, and runs events, seminars and workshops to grow and encourage conversations around mental health.

The LBC also runs the mental health training programmes BarberTalk, Hair&BeautyTalk and a non-industry-specific version called HereToTalk. All the training programmes are endorsed by Habia (Hair and Beauty Industry Authority – recognized by the UK government as a standard-setting body for the hair industry) and recognized on their Continuing Professional Development (CPD) programme.

The charity regularly partners with college hair and beauty departments, which become "Lions Academies", ensuring mental health is a topic on the curriculum. They ensure that all students are aware of mental wellbeing and take, at least, the BarberTalk Lite training programme.

In 2021, the LBC opened their first Lions Barbers, a non-profit barbers' shop in London whose profits are donated to the Lions Barber Collective to be spent on working toward their vision of a world free from suicide.

Find out more at www.thelionsbarbercollective.com.

ABOUT US

Welbeck Balance publishes books dedicated to changing lives. Our mission is to deliver life enhancing books to help improve your wellbeing so that you can live your life with greater clarity and meaning, wherever you are on life's journey. Our Trigger books are specifically devoted to opening up conversations about mental health and wellbeing.

Welbeck Balance and Trigger are part of the Welbeck Publishing Group – a globally recognized independent publisher based in London. Welbeck are renowned for our innovative ideas, production values and developing long-lasting content. Our books have been translated into over 30 languages in more than 60 countries around the world.

If you love books, then join the club and sign up to our newsletter for exclusive offers, extracts, author interviews and more information.

www.welbeckpublishing.com   www.triggerhub.org

🐦 welbeckpublish   🐦 Triggercalm
📷 welbeckpublish   📷 Triggercalm
🅕 welbeckuk   🅕 Triggercalm

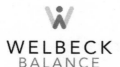

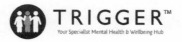